Understanding
Thyroid Problems

Bryan McIver M.D., Ph.D.
Anthony Toft M.D.

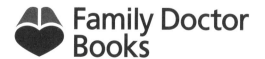

IMPORTANT NOTICE

This book is not intended as a substitute for personal
medical advice but as a supplement to that advice for
the patient who wishes to understand more
about his/her condition.

Before starting, stopping or changing any form of
treatment YOU SHOULD ALWAYS CONSULT
YOUR MEDICAL PRACTITIONER.

In particular you should note that advances in medical
science occur rapidly and some of the information about
drugs and treatment contained in this booklet may
very soon be out of date.

© Family Doctor Publications 2006

ISBN-10: 1-4285-0003-0
ISBN-13: 978-1-4285-0003-7

Contents

About the authors

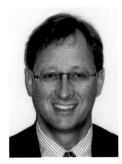

Dr. Bryan McIver M.D.
Is a Consultant in Endocrinology, Metabolism and Nutrition at the Mayo Clinic in Rochester, Minnesota. He has extensive experience treating patients with diseases of the thyroid. He also runs a research lab, working on thyroid cancer genetics and on new treatments for patients with thyroid cancer. He is the Chairman of the Thyroid Group within the Division of Endocrinology at Mayo Clinic, a group of over 40 full time Endocrine specialists.

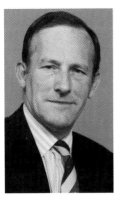

Anthony Toft CBE, M.D., FRCP
Is a Consultant Physician and Endocrinologist at the Royal Infirmary of Edinburgh where he specializes in the diagnosis and management of patients with thyroid disease. Dr. Toft has been President of the British Thyroid Association and President of the Royal College of Physicians of Edinburgh.

Introduction

What is the thyroid gland?
The thyroid gland is a small fleshy organ, which lies in the front of the neck just under the skin, below the "Adam's apple" (larynx) and in front of the windpipe (trachea). The thyroid consists of two lobes, one on the right and one on the left, joined by a bridge across the middle (the isthmus); each lobe measures around two and a half inches long, the entire gland weighing less than one ounce. Despite its small size, it is a very important gland, because it makes thyroid hormone, a chemical that controls metabolism and is needed for the normal working of every cell in the body.

Thyroid hormones
The thyroid gland actually makes two forms of thyroid hormone: thyroxine [thy-rox-een] (also known as T_4) and triiodothyronine [tri-iodo-thyro-neen] (shortened to T_3). These hormones are released into the bloodstream where they circulate around the body and have their effects.

Iodine is an essential part of these hormones, which cannot be made properly if iodine is lacking in the diet.

Thyroid gland

The thyroid gland lies in the neck between the skin and the voice box (larynx). The thyroid gland is a butterfly-shaped gland consisting of two lobes, one on each side of the trachea (windpipe).

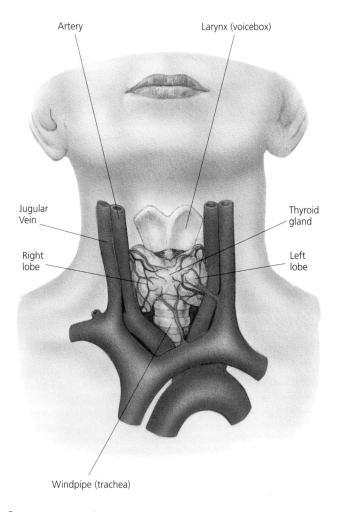

There are four atoms of iodine in each molecule of thyroxine, leading to the abbreviation T_4, and three atoms of iodine in each molecule of T_3.

Although the thyroid gland produces both T_4 and T_3, most of the hormone released by the gland is in the form of T_4. T_4 is not itself an active hormone, however, and only becomes active when it is converted—mostly by the liver and kidneys—into T_3, a process that involves the removal of one of the atoms of iodine. This complicated system may be one of the means by which the body's level of thyroid hormone is very carefully and precisely regulated.

The importance of iodine

Although iodine is needed to make thyroid hormone, it is not present naturally in large amounts in most food. For this reason, iodine is added to a wide variety of foods in the USA, including salt, flour, and baked goods. Seafood (though not fish caught in inland lakes and streams) is naturally high in iodine and is a good source of dietary iodine.

Most multivitamin preparations also contain the full US recommended daily allowance (RDA) of iodine, 150 mcg (micrograms) daily. During the 1800s and early 1900s, iodine deficiency was common in the USA—particularly in the mid-western and mountain states—but iodine added to salt and flour has made iodine deficiency in the US very rare nowadays.

However, people in other parts of the world, including parts of Africa, Asia, and South America, continue to suffer from the effects of iodine deficiency, causing needless disease and suffering.

If there is not enough iodine for the thyroid gland to make T_3 and T_4, the thyroid gland grows larger to

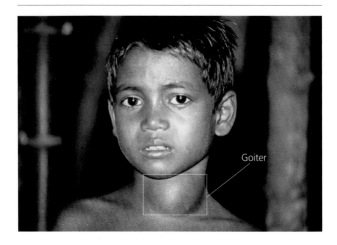

Goiter

compensate, causing a goiter (an enlarged thyroid, see page 84), and an underactive thyroid (hypothyroidism, see page 51).

Worldwide, iodine deficiency remains a leading cause of mental retardation, caused by hypothyroidism during pregnancy. Too much iodine can also cause thyroid problems, however, and may cause the thyroid gland to produce too much thyroid hormone (hyperthyroidism, see page 10), or trigger inflammation of the gland (Hashimoto's disease, see page 51).

Balancing the hormones
In healthy people, the levels of T_3 and T_4 in the blood are controlled within a narrow normal range by a hormone known as thyroid-stimulating hormone (TSH). TSH is produced by the pituitary gland, a small gland that lies beneath the brain, just behind the bridge of the nose.

If thyroid hormone levels in the blood begin to fall, the pituitary senses the problem and increases TSH

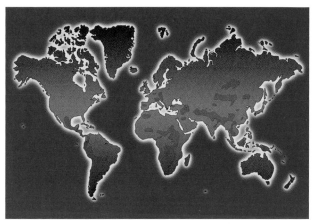

The red areas on this world map show the regions of the world in which iodine-deficiency goiter remains a common disorder. This occurs largely because the soil, and consequently locally produced food, lacks sufficient iodine.

production which, in turn, stimulates the thyroid gland to make more thyroid hormone.

If thyroid hormone levels in the blood increase, the pituitary makes less TSH, so turning down the activity of the thyroid gland. This control of the thyroid gland by the pituitary gland is known as "negative feedback," and provides very stable levels of T_4 and T_3 in the bloodstream of healthy people.

The level of TSH in the blood indicates how hard the pituitary wants the thyroid to work; as a result, measuring the TSH level is a very accurate way to determine whether the thyroid gland is working normally.

For people receiving treatment for a thyroid condition, the TSH level is also an excellent way to determine whether the treatment is working.

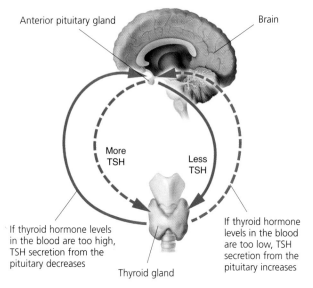

The production of thyroid hormones by the thyroid gland is regulated by the pituitary gland, which produces thyroid-stimulating hormone (TSH) in response to the levels of thyroid hormones in the blood.

Hypothyroidism and hyperthyroidism

If your physician suspects that you have a thyroid problem (hypothyroidism or hyperthyroidism), he or she will send a blood sample to the laboratory for measurement of the TSH.

A high level of TSH indicates that the thyroid is underactive (hypothyroid), while a low level of TSH suggests that the thyroid is overactive (hyperthyroid). In most cases, the diagnosis will also be confirmed by measuring the levels of T_4 and sometimes T_3 in the blood, as well as a number of more complicated tests, discussed throughout this book.

In most cases, the TSH level alone is a very accurate

test of thyroid function, but like all tests, there are times when it can be misleading. While these times are rare, it is important not to rely too heavily on any single test, if symptoms suggest that a thyroid problem exists.

Thyroid disease is common. Hypothyroidism, hyperthyroidism, enlargement of the gland (goiter), or thyroid nodules affect as many as one in 20 people in the US, particularly people of northern European or Asian ancestry, though other ethnic groups can also be affected.

Many of these patients remain undiagnosed, because thyroid testing is not part of a "routine physical" in most parts of the USA, and because the symptoms of thyroid disease may resemble many other conditions, or simply be felt to be part of "getting older."

Although few physicians believe that routine screening for thyroid disease is justified for everyone in the USA, patients who show any symptoms of thyroid disease should certainly be offered testing.

Certain groups of people at particularly high risk for the development of thyroid disease (for example, women over the age of 35, men and women over 60–65 years, people with a family history of thyroid disease) should also be offered thyroid screening.

Various recommendations have been made by a number of professional groups, including the American College of Physicians, the American Thyroid Association, the Endocrine Society, and the American Association of Clinical Endocrinologists, and those recommendations do not always agree with one another.

The most important factor is to discuss the possibility of thyroid disease with your own physician to determine whether testing the thyroid is necessary and worthwhile for you.

Thyroid disease of all types is more common in women than in men (about 3 to 1), and often runs in families—most often through the women of the family—so that family screening may be worthwhile. In some cases, there may be a link between the development of thyroid disease and other medical conditions such as diabetes, pernicious anemia, and inflammatory diseases, including rheumatoid arthritis and lupus.

Fortunately, most thyroid diseases can be successfully treated, though treatment and monitoring may be needed for the rest of the patient's life. Even thyroid cancer, which is fortunately rare, can be treated and often cured, if it is detected early enough and treated appropriately.

In most cases of hypothyroidism, a family physician or internist will be able to diagnose, treat, and monitor the condition accurately. Most patients with hyperthyroidism, unexplained goiter, or thyroid growths, nodules, or thyroid cancer should be referred to an endocrinologist, a specialist in disorders of the thyroid and other glands.

The remaining chapters in this book deal with each of the most common thyroid disorders. Additional information can be found in a number of sources, including books, informational leaflets, internet sites, and technical documents, some of which are listed in the Useful Addresses section at the end of this book.

However, the most important source of information for anyone diagnosed with a thyroid condition is their own physician or endocrinologist. It is important to remember that the information in this book should only be used as a guide, and never as a substitute for the advice of a fully trained physician.

KEY POINTS

■ The thyroid gland makes thyroid hormone, which is essential for normal health

■ Too much or too little iodine can trigger thyroid disease

■ Thyroid disease is common, affecting around one in 20 people

■ More women than men are affected

■ Your physician can diagnose most common thyroid diseases, using a simple blood test

■ Treatment is usually successful, but treatment and monitoring may be required for the rest of the patient's life

Overactive thyroid (Hyperthyroidism)

Graves' disease

An overactive thyroid gland (hyperthyroidism, also known as thyrotoxicosis) is caused by the release of too much T_4 and T_3 from the thyroid gland. There are several causes of this condition, but the most common are Graves' disease—seen most often in women between the ages of 30 and 50 years—and "toxic multinodular goiter," which typically affects adults over 50 years old. Other, less common causes of hyperthyroidism are mentioned briefly at the end of this chapter.

Graves' disease is by far the most common cause of an overactive thyroid, responsible for over three-quarters of cases. The disease is named for an Irish physician, Dr. Robert Graves, who first described the condition in detail over 200 years ago.

Although it is most common in women, the condition also affects men, who can sometimes be affected more severely. The most common age at which Graves' disease is diagnosed is between 30 and

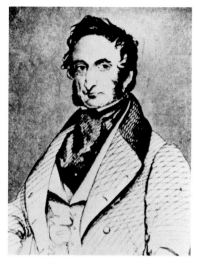

Robert Graves, 1796–1853

50 years, but there are many cases of teenagers or children being affected, and it remains a frequent cause of hyperthyroidism, even in old age.

Most of the symptoms of Graves' disease are caused by the production of too much thyroid hormone, which causes a wide array of symptoms affecting many systems in the body. Those symptoms are discussed in detail below (page 15).

In Graves' disease, the symptoms can have a wide range of severity from almost non-existent to extremely severe, and in a small number of cases, the problem can even be life-threatening. Fortunately, with proper diagnosis and treatment, the condition is almost always treatable, though it may not be curable.

Graves' disease is caused by the immune system making an antibody that stimulates the thyroid gland. This antibody circulates in the blood, where it can often be detected in laboratory tests (TSH receptor antibodies, thyroid-stimulating antibodies, TSI or TRAb). When the antibody reaches the thyroid gland, the gland responds by becoming more active, producing too much thyroid hormone. The thyroid gland may become larger in response to the stimulation, causing a goiter, which may be felt in the neck or, in some cases, become visible to the naked eye.

The cause of the stimulating antibody production is not known, though a genetic tendency and an infectious trigger are suspected. Certainly, patients with Graves' disease often have a family history of thyroid problems or of other inflammatory problems, suggesting that there may be a genetic cause. Severe stress—the loss of a loved one, for example—which may alter immune system function, is also thought to play a role in triggering some cases of Graves' disease.

Graves' disease is one of a group of diseases known as "autoimmune disease," in which the immune system is triggered to attack parts of the normal body. Other autoimmune diseases include Type 1 diabetes (young-onset diabetes), pernicious anemia (deficiency of vitamin B_{12}), myasthenia gravis (weakness of various muscles), and failure of the adrenal glands (Addison's disease).

Patients with Graves' disease are at somewhat increased risk for these conditions, though fortunately, most people with Graves' disease do not develop them. There is also an increased risk of other immune system-related conditions, including celiac disease (gluten sensitivity, an intestinal allergy to dietary gluten), rheumatoid arthritis, lupus, in which multiple organs are affected by inflammation, and a variety of other rare inflammatory diseases.

Each of these conditions is caused by the immune system treating specific parts of the body as something foreign, and making an effort to destroy or "reject" those normal organs.

In the case of Grave's disease, that "rejection" leads to the formation of antibodies that actually stimulate, rather than weaken, the gland, causing it to become overactive. The cause of this immune system abnormality remains unknown, though a great deal of research is being done on this subject.

At the time of writing, treatment for these autoimmune conditions is focused on treating the effects of the disease, not its cause. Treatment that damps down the immune system (immuno-suppression) can be potentially dangerous, increasing the chances of infection and possibly cancers of various types—the treatment could be worse than the disease!

As we gain a better understanding of the causes of diseases such as Graves' disease, this situation may change, allowing better, safer, and more effective treatment in the future.

In addition to an overactive thyroid, some patients with Graves' disease also develop swelling and prominence of the eyes (exophthalmos, proptosis, or Graves' ophthalmopathy), which is discussed in more detail later (page 42).

A few patients also suffer from raised, swollen, red, itchy areas of skin on the front of the lower legs or on the top of the feet, known as pretibial myxedema.

Each of these conditions is caused by the same abnormality of the immune system that triggers the overactive thyroid. Treatment of the overactive thyroid may help to "cool down" the immune system, helping with these other problems too, but sometimes the eye and skin problems need treatment in their own right, if they fail to settle after the thyroid gland has been treated.

Toxic multinodular goiter

The second most common cause of hyperthyroidism is the development of an enlarged, nodular (lumpy) thyroid, known as a multinodular goiter. Typically, this form of goiter develops gradually and progressively over many years or decades, and eventually causes worsening hyperthyroidism (known as toxic multinodular goiter (TMNG) or Plummer's disease, named after Dr. Henry S. Plummer, of the Mayo Clinic). Hyperthyroidism of this type usually develops gradually, and may escape detection for a long time.

Most patients with TMNG are older adults, often over 70 years old, though patients may sometimes be as young as 40. Often, there is a family history of goiter, so presumably there is again a genetic background to this disease.

In the case of TMNG, unlike in Graves' disease, however, there does not seem to be any relationship to the immune system, and the gland is not driven to enlarge or become overactive by any known trigger, except, perhaps, a history of iodine deficiency in childhood.

Once the gland begins to enlarge, the condition tends to progress slowly over many years, and there is nothing that seems to prevent that progression. In particular, supplements of iodine or thyroid hormone, which have been used in the past in an effort to shrink the goiter, do not prevent the slow worsening of the disease. Indeed, excessive intake of iodine, like gasoline on a campfire, may actually make the hyperthyroidism worse, by providing the gland with the fuel from which to make excess thyroid hormone.

Once again, effective treatment is available for TMNG, though typically that treatment is only used once the gland has become overactive, unless the goiter is large enough to cause local symptoms in the neck, including difficulty swallowing, breathing problems, voice changes, or pressure symptoms.

What is the pattern of development?

The onset of symptoms of hyperthyroidism may be slow, insidious, and barely noticeable, for example in patients with a slowly progressive TMNG, or they can be abrupt, dramatic, and severe, especially in young people with severe Graves' disease.

In retrospect, most patients have had symptoms for at least six months before they see their physician. Not all patients with hyperthyroidism will have all the symptoms listed below, and of course, these symptoms can sometimes be caused by other conditions.

Symptoms of an overactive thyroid gland

When considering the symptoms of thyroid disease, it is important not simply to use these symptoms as a "checklist." Instead, the overall pattern of symptoms, their severity, and the speed of onset should be combined with the findings on examination to determine whether a thyroid condition is likely to be present.

In elderly people, in particular, the classic symptoms may be partly or completely absent, with the patient suffering symptoms more suggestive of depression or "old age." It is this problem that leads many endocrinologists to suggest that a routine physical in older patients should include thyroid testing.

Weight loss and hunger

High levels of T_4 and T_3 speed up the metabolism, causing increased energy use, which burns calories. Most patients with hyperthyroidism experience some weight loss, from just a few pounds in mild cases, to as much as 50 or 60 pounds in severe cases.

The appetite is stimulated too, however, so a few patients—particularly those with only a slightly overactive thyroid—may not actually experience any weight loss, or may even notice a few pounds of weight gain.

Hunger is a common effect of hyperthyroidism, and in extreme cases, that hunger can be bad enough to cause the patient to have to eat additional meals, or even to wake up at night to eat.

Patients who lose weight because of hyperthyroidism may be tempted to believe that easy weight loss (no need for a diet or exercise!) is a beneficial side effect of their condition. A few patients with otherwise mild symptoms may even try to avoid treatment for their thyroid, fearing that the weight will return.

Unfortunately, hyperthyroidism is neither safe nor, ultimately, effective as a treatment for weight loss. The weight loss caused by excess thyroid hormone causes muscle loss more than loss of fat. Ultimately, that muscle loss slows the basal metabolic rate (muscle burns many more calories than fat, even at rest), and the weight loss stops.

Once the hyperthyroidism is treated, the metabolism returns to normal and the change in body composition (less muscle and more fat) causes a lower than normal metabolic rate. And now the weight starts to rise.

The weakened muscles are harder to rebuild, slowing recovery and encouraging the accumulation of more fat. In the meantime, the stimulated appetite continues to drive an increased consumption of high-calorie foods, which accelerates the problem.

Delaying or avoiding treatment for an overactive thyroid may actually worsen the eventual outcome, at least as far as the weight regain is concerned, and certainly increases the risk of other adverse effects of the overactive thyroid.

Heat intolerance and sweating

As the metabolic rate increases, the body produces excess heat, which it then gets rid of by opening the blood vessels in the skin and by sweating. This leads to both a feeling of heat and easily triggered sweating.

Amongst women who have experienced menopause, the symptoms may resemble a return of menopausal hot flashes and night sweats. Younger women may also wonder whether they are starting an early menopause, particularly because hyperthyroidism may affect the menstrual period too.

Typical symptoms include feeling excessively hot in warm weather or with central heating, preferring cool weather and air-conditioning turned up high, and feeling comfortable dressed lightly, even in the winter.

In extreme cases, the inability to tolerate heat may lead to disagreements with friends and family, because you are constantly turning down the thermostat, opening windows in cold weather, or throwing blankets off the bed at night.

Irritability and poor concentration

You may find yourself increasingly unable to cope with the stresses of normal day-to-day life, including work, caring for children, and dealing with friends and family. You may lose your temper more often than usual, find yourself abnormally sensitive to criticism, and experiencing emotional instability, perhaps bursting into tears or exploding into a rage for no apparent reason.

Anxiety is common and full-blown panic attacks may also occur. You may find it difficult to focus and concentrate, which can adversely affect your performance at school, college, or work. Tasks requiring intense concentration may become more difficult, and there is a tendency to become less well organized than usual, jumping from one task to another.

Sleep disturbance and altered energy levels

Hyperthyroidism acts on the brain in a way that is similar to an overdose of caffeine, initially creating a feeling of extra energy. With very mild hyperthyroidism, this can be felt as a benefit, but any benefit quickly gives way to disrupted sleep, an inescapable feeling of useless energy, and the sensation of being unable to rest or even to sit still.

It often results in worsening fatigue or even exhaustion, partly because of sleep deprivation. This symptom worsens the irritability, emotional instability, and lack of concentration that also come from hyperthyroidism.

Palpitations

Most patients experience palpitations—an awareness of the heartbeat—and many feel a more rapid than normal heart rate. Particularly at night, the forceful contractions of the heart can be disturbing or frightening.

Extra heart beats (premature ventricular contractions or PVCs) are common, and may be noticed as a "skipped beat," because of the delay before the next normal heart beat. Among older patients, or in severe, long-standing hyperthyroidism even in younger people, an irregular rapid heartbeat, known as atrial fibrillation, may develop.

Atrial fibrillation can be a serious complication of hyperthyroidism, which can cause heart failure or a stroke, and must often be treated with blood thinners to prevent blood clots (coumadin), and drugs to slow or control the heart rate (digoxin, beta-blockers). After correction of the hyperthyroidism, the heartbeat may return to normal, or may require either electrical treatment (cardioversion) or continued drug treatment.

Shortness of breath
This is most likely to be noticeable during and after exertion, for example, after climbing a flight of stairs. Patients with asthma may find their condition made worse by hyperthyroidism.

Tremor
Most patients complain of shaky hands, and a feeling of tremulousness. This can be mistaken for anxiety or, in older patients, Parkinson's disease.

Muscle weakness
Often, the thigh muscles, in particular, become weak, making it hard to stand up from a sitting position, or

to climb stairs. Muscle weakness may also lead to loss of balance, a particular concern for older patients. This muscle loss, typically, is a sign of severe or long-standing hyperthyroidism.

Frequent bowel motions
There is often an increase in their frequency of bowel motions as well as a tendency toward looser stools, causing a softer than normal stool two, three, or even more times daily. Diarrhea can sometimes be a problem.

Altered menstrual function
The menstrual cycle may become irregular and periods lighter than usual. The period may even disappear completely until the hyperthyroidism is adequately treated. Fertility is reduced and it may be difficult for a woman to conceive during hyperthyroidism.

Skin, hair and nail changes
The skin becomes more sensitive, may be itchy, and is much more likely to develop hives (urticaria) in response to minor allergies. You may find that the whole body itches, which can be a very troublesome symptom.

The hair may become thinner and finer than usual. It is common for a hairdresser or beautician to notice these changes. The nails may also become brittle, lift easily from the nail bed, and become split or ridged.

However, patients with Graves' disease may rarely develop raised, swollen, red, itchy patches on their lower legs and feet (pretibial myxedema), which can be difficult to treat, and may not resolve with treatment of the thyroid.

Following treatment of hyperthyroidism, the rapid fall in the level of thyroid hormone can trigger a sudden and sometimes startling loss of hair, known as *telogen effluvium* (a Latin term meaning "a river of hair"), which is most often seen within 4–6 weeks of the treatment. Although the hair loss can be dramatic, this condition does not cause baldness and is always followed by a re-growth of healthy normal hair. It simply reflects the abrupt change in the hormone levels in the blood, and may be seen in several other conditions that cause sudden hormonal shifts—most frequently in women following a pregnancy.

A much less common cause of hair loss can also affect a small number of patients with Graves' disease. *Alopecia areata,* which causes patchy areas of true baldness, is another of the autoimmune conditions that can sometimes be seen in association with Graves' disease, although the thyroid disease itself—and treatment of the thyroid—has no impact on the condition.

In the case of *alopecia areata,* the immune attack seems to be focused on the hair follicle. Treatment for this condition may include injected steroids and hair growth stimulants, and should be guided by a dermatologist.

Bone loss and osteoporosis

Hyperthyroidism accelerates the loss of bone that often affects women past menopause. Untreated, this can lead to an increased risk of fractures.

Goiter

Although a goiter may be visible in the neck, and will almost always be palpable in cases of hyperthyroidism, it is unlikely that the goiter will cause any symptoms.

Occasionally, however, large multinodular goiters cause a sensation of fullness in the neck, and large goiters can also cause difficulty with swallowing, changes in the voice and—very rarely—breathing difficulty.

Goiters causing hyperthyroidism are almost never tender or painful, so the presence of a painful swelling in the neck may point to some other disease process requiring evaluation.

Eye symptoms

Changes in the eyes may occur in some patients with Graves' disease, but do not occur in other causes of an overactive thyroid. Problems experienced by patients with Graves' disease can include excessive watering, made worse by wind and bright light, pain, dryness and grittiness, double vision (which goes away with one eye closed), and blurring of vision.

Swelling of the tissues around the eyes, redness, and prominence of the eye caused by retraction of the upper eyelid are also seen.

Some patients develop true protrusion of the eye (exophthalmos or proptosis), caused by an increase in the pressure behind the eyeball, pushing the eye forward.

These symptoms can be very troublesome, and in rare cases may be severe enough that the eyesight can be threatened. Evaluation by an experienced ophthalmologist, working in conjunction with an endocrinologist, may be necessary. A more detailed discussion of Graves Eye Disease begins on page 42.

Confirming the diagnosis
Blood test

If symptoms point to an overactive thyroid, your physician will want to confirm the diagnosis, by sending a blood sample to the lab for a TSH measurement. An overactive thyroid will cause the TSH level to be low. In most cases, measurement of the T_4 or T_3 levels in

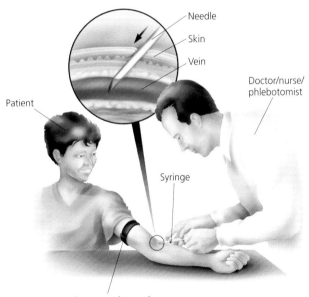

Needle

Skin

Vein

Doctor/nurse/ phlebotomist

Patient

Syringe

A tourniquet may be used to make the vein more prominent

For a blood test a vein is chosen and the blood draw site cleaned. A hollow needle attached to a syringe is inserted into the vein and blood drawn out for testing.

the blood allows your doctor to determine just how active the thyroid really is. Measurement of the antibody levels in the same blood sample can help confirm whether the problem is Graves' disease, TMNG, or one of the other, less common, causes of hyperthyroidism.

Thyroid scan and uptake

Two additional tests are frequently used to determine why the thyroid has become overactive and how it might be treated. These tests are a thyroid scan and an "uptake" measurement, which may be performed separately or at the same time.

These tests both involve the use of radioactive "tracers," in which a tiny dose of radioactive iodine or a tracer called technetium is given either by mouth (for the radioactive iodine) or by injection into a vein (for technetium).

Scans of this type are usually performed by specialists in nuclear medicine and take place in a hospital or large medical center, to which your physician will refer you. The dose of iodine used is so small that it can even be given to someone who is known to be allergic to iodine.

It is important to realize that the radioactive iodine used in these scans is much weaker than the radioactive iodine that may be used to treat some patients with an overactive thyroid, and will have no effect on the function of the thyroid gland. The amount of radiation in each of these tracers is tiny, and carries no known risk to the patient or to others around him or her.

You should always inform your physician, however, if you are pregnant, may be pregnant, or if you are

Thyroid scan

Isotope scanning uses a gamma camera to create a picture from radiation emitted from the body after a radioactive isotope, such as technetium-99m, has been injected.

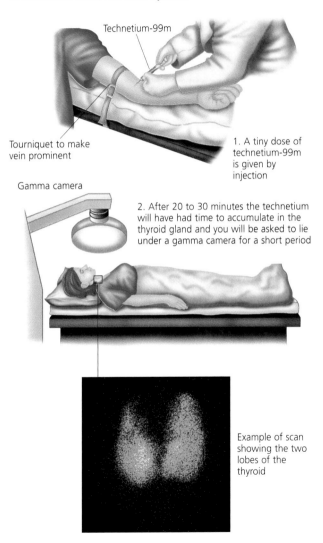

Technetium-99m

Tourniquet to make vein prominent

1. A tiny dose of technetium-99m is given by injection

Gamma camera

2. After 20 to 30 minutes the technetium will have had time to accumulate in the thyroid gland and you will be asked to lie under a gamma camera for a short period

Example of scan showing the two lobes of the thyroid

breast-feeding, because most specialists avoid the use of radioactive tracers in those circumstances.

The "uptake," which can be measured 4 hours, 6 hours, or 24 hours after the radioactive iodine is given (depending on the type of radiation used), helps to determine just how active the gland is, and whether radioactive iodine in higher doses could be used to treat the hyperthyroidism.

The scan, in which a picture is taken of the thyroid gland, allows the doctor to assess whether the entire gland is overactive, or whether the problem is that one or more nodules within the gland have become overactive.

If a nodule is found, either by examination or during the scan, further evaluation may be needed before treatment for the hyperthyroidism is started. Evaluation of thyroid nodules is discussed in the chapter on Thyroid Nodules (page 94).

Treatment for hyperthyroidism

Three forms of treatment are available for hyperthyroidism caused by Graves' disease or TMNG, including:

- Medication
- Surgery
- Radioactive iodine

Each of these treatments has advantages and disadvantages, and each has some risks as well as benefits. None of these options is perfect, but each can be effective and safe. It is important to realize that there is no one "best" treatment for every patient. The decision as to which treatment you receive should be made only after you have had a chance to discuss each one of these fully with an endocrinologist or other physician experienced in the management of hyperthyroidism.

Once the diagnosis of hyperthyroidism is made, your symptoms may be improved by taking a beta-blocker drug such as propranolol (Inderal™), atenolol (Tenormin™) or metoprolol (Toprol™). These drugs partially counteract the actions of thyroid hormone, and can ease at least some of the symptoms, although they do not treat the thyroid problem itself.

They are useful only for short-term symptom relief. Beta-blocker drugs should be used cautiously by people with diabetes, low blood pressure, asthma, or chronic obstructive pulmonary disease (COPD). Typically, beta-blockers are prescribed only for a few weeks, until the hyperthyroidism is controlled by one of the following treatments.

Antithyroid drugs

Antithyroid drugs work by blocking the thyroid from using iodine to make thyroid hormone. The drugs are taken by mouth between one and three times daily, the dose being adjusted to return the thyroid hormone levels to normal.

The most commonly used antithyroid drugs in North America are propylthiouracil (PTU for short) and methimazole (sometimes abbreviated to MMZ), though carbimazole (CBZ) is also sometimes used. Each of these drugs reduces the amount of thyroid hormone made by the thyroid gland. PTU is available in 50-milligram (mg) tablets, while MMZ and CBZ come in strengths of 5 mg and 20 mg. One tablet of PTU (50 mg) has roughly the same effect on the thyroid as one 5 mg tablet of MMZ or CBZ. A high dose (6 to 9 tablets daily) is used initially to bring the thyroid under control.

Symptoms of hyperthyroidism usually start to improve within 10 to 14 days, and the blood tests start to show improvement after 2–4 weeks. Following this, the endocrinologist will usually be able to reduce the dose gradually down to 1 or 2 tablets daily (usually taken as a single daily dose), depending upon the results of measurements of your blood levels of TSH, T_4, and T_3.

Some endocrinologists prefer to use a high dose of PTZU or MMZ throughout the course of treatment. Because this would eventually cause you to develop an underactive thyroid gland, thyroxine (thyroid hormone tablets) is added to the antithyroid drug once thyroid hormone levels have returned to normal.

The advantage of this type of treatment is that it may not need to be reviewed so often. However, this approach is no more effective in controlling hyperthyroidism than smaller doses of the antithyroid drugs alone, and careful follow-up of patients taking these drugs is essential no matter what medication is prescribed for them.

Follow-up usually requires blood tests every 3 months and a visit to an endocrinologist every three to six months throughout the course of treatment. The full course of treatment usually lasts between 12 and 18 months, after which time the drug is withdrawn and the blood tested at intervals again to ensure the hyperthyroidism does not recur.

Antithyroid drugs work in almost everyone who takes them in a high enough dosage. Unfortunately, hyperthyroidism recurs in more than 50% of patients

How antithyroid drugs work

Antithyroid drugs interfere with the manufacture of thyroid hormones, bringing the high levels found in hyperthyroidism back to normal.

Before drug
Thyroid gland is over-producing thyroid hormones

After drug
Thyroid hormone levels restored to normal

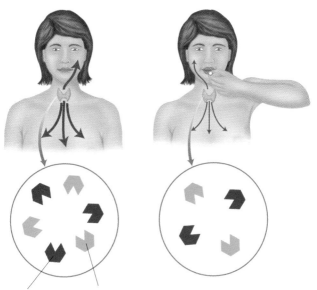

Thyroxine (T_4)   Triiodothyronine (T_3)

with Graves' disease who have successfully completed a course of these drugs. If the hyperthyroidism does recur—usually within the first year or two—one of the alternative treatments is usually recommended to prevent the problem from coming back again in the future.

Because these drugs do not treat the cause of hyperthyroidism in TMNG, almost all patients with this type of hyperthyroidism develop hyperthyroidism again when the drugs are withdrawn. For this reason, patients with TMNG are rarely treated this way.

Side effects of drugs

Like all drugs, PTU and MMZ have side effects. The most common side effect is a bad taste after taking the tablet. This can be controlled by taking the tablet with a meal. Most people find this side effect to be nothing more than a minor inconvenience.

An allergic reaction causing a skin rash (hives) affects two percent of patients who take these drugs. Hives form an itchy, raised, red, bumpy skin rash, which tends to cover the whole body. The medical term for this condition is urticaria; it is like the rash you get from contact with poison ivy.

If you develop urticaria while taking these drugs, you should stop taking them and inform your doctor. The rash will disappear within a few days, during which time the itch can be relieved by antihistamine tablets.

Abnormal liver test results may occur in a small number of patients taking PTU or MMZ, particularly in high doses in the first few weeks of treatment. The problem usually disappears when the dose is reduced, though occasionally the drug must be withdrawn if the liver is seriously affected. The liver almost always recovers fully after the dose is reduced or the drug is stopped.

The most serious side effect of antithyroid drugs is a reduction in the number of white blood cells (agranulocytosis), which can make you prone to a bacterial infection. This shows itself as a very sore throat—similar to strep throat—with canker sores (aphthous ulcers) and a high fever.

Agranulocytosis is a medical emergency and you must contact your physician *immediately* if it happens, and arrange to have a CBC (complete blood count) checked. If, for any reason, you cannot reach your own physician or your endocrinologist, you should immediately attend an emergency room or trauma center and explain that you need this test done—take this book along with you to show this section to the ER doctor, if necessary!

If the white cell count is normal or high, the problem is not the result of the drugs, and your sore throat should be treated in the normal way. If the white cell count is low, however, the PTU or MMZ should be stopped, and you will probably need to take antibiotics and may even be admitted to hospital for a short period, for monitoring.

Fortunately this serious side effect of antithyroid drugs is rare, affecting fewer than 1 in 300 to 1 in 500 patients. The white cell count always recovers, after the right treatment.

Other rare side effects include aching joints and stiffness, nausea and headache. Once again, these side effects are generally temporary and improve or disappear once the drug is stopped.

Surgery

Surgery to remove the thyroid—or most of the thyroid—was the first effective treatment for Graves' disease, and it remains a good treatment to this day, though it is certainly now the least popular of the three treatment options.

The goal of the surgery is to remove most of the thyroid gland, so that it can no longer produce too much thyroid hormone. It is not necessary to remove

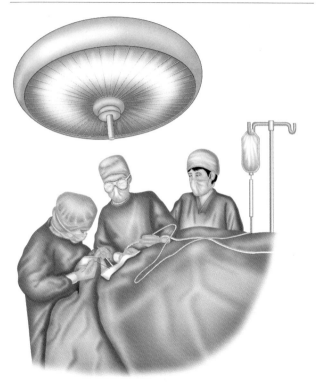

Surgery may be the treatment of choice particularly for a young patient with Graves' disease and a large goiter.

the entire gland, however, and leaving a small amount of the thyroid behind allows the surgeon to protect the other important structures in the neck, reducing the risks of surgery.

Surgery on the thyroid gland is usually performed either by a specialized endocrine surgeon, or by an otorhinolaryngologist (ear, nose, and throat surgeon). Whoever performs the surgery should certainly be experienced operating in this area, and it is usual for the surgeon and the endocrinologist to work closely together to prepare a patient for this type of surgery.

Before the surgery is performed, the thyroid hormone levels in your blood should be returned to normal. That is usually achieved by a short course of antithyroid drugs, followed by an iodine-containing medication for 10 to 14 days before surgery. This treatment is not radioactive, and simply helps to reduce the size of the thyroid gland and its blood flow, making the job technically easier for the surgeon.

Surgery usually lasts between 1 and 2 hours, with a total hospital stay of 24 to 36 hours, unless complications develop. Patients are usually discharged from hospital after already taking replacement thyroid hormone, and follow-up for the thyroid hormone levels is performed in the same way as for treatment of an underactive thyroid (see hypothyroidism, page 51).

What you should know about surgery

Surgery leaves a scar, usually two or three inches long, low at the front of the neck. This scar can be prominent at first, but usually becomes pale and barely noticeable after a few months. In many cases it is almost invisible within a year.

In rare cases (less than one percent), the parathyroid glands, that lie close to the thyroid and control the level of calcium in the blood, may be damaged. In such cases, long-term treatment with a strong dose of vitamin D and a high dose of calcium becomes necessary.

Equally rare is damage to one of the nerves controlling the larynx (the voice box), known as the recurrent laryngeal nerves. These nerves lie immediately behind the thyroid, and surgery on the gland can stretch, bruise, or (in very rare cases) sever these nerves.

Damage to the nerves can cause a significant change in the quality of the voice, with hoarseness and raspiness. Unless the nerve is actually completely cut—a very rare event—the voice will gradually return to normal in most cases. However, fear of this complication is one reason why surgery is a less appealing option for some people with hyperthyroidism, singers in particular.

Surgery is very effective in treating hyperthyroidism caused both by Graves' disease and TMNG. Almost all patients will be cured immediately, though many patients will develop an underactive thyroid instead, requiring long-term treatment with thyroid hormone (see hypothyroidism, page 51).

A recurrence of hyperthyroidism is possible, sometimes many years after thyroid surgery, because the remaining thyroid tissue can be stimulated to grow over time. However, this is a very uncommon event with modern surgery.

Surgery remains the fastest and most certain way to eliminate hyperthyroidism, caused either by Graves' disease or by TMNG. Although it is chosen by only a small number of patients, it remains an excellent choice for some people.

Radioactive iodine (iodine-131)

Treatment with radioactive iodine is being used more and more frequently in the US to treat patients with hyperthyroidism, because it is highly effective, relatively inexpensive, and appears to be very safe. It is also very convenient, usually requiring only a single dose to cure the problem.

Because the thyroid gland uses iodine to make thyroid hormone (see page 1), hyperthyroidism causes the gland to take up a large amount of iodine. In fact, among patients with Graves' disease, as much as 80–90% or more of a dose of iodine taken by mouth is absorbed into the thyroid gland within 24 hours.

If the iodine is made radioactive, that radioactivity is concentrated in the gland, causing injury to and even destruction of the gland. Over the course of a few weeks, the gland weakens, shrinks, and is reabsorbed by the body.

In the meantime, the thyroid hormone levels fall from the high levels seen in hyperthyroidism, to normal. In most cases, the hormone levels then continue to fall to below the normal range and the patient develops an underactive thyroid (hypothyroidism, see page 51).

Fortunately, hypothyroidism is quite easy to treat, using thyroid hormone, which is taken by mouth once each day. Because this is an expected outcome of treatment with radioactive iodine, most patients are diagnosed quickly and they only suffer the symptoms of hypothyroidism transiently.

Radioactive iodine is taken by mouth in the form of a capsule or a liquid that tastes like water. It is usually administered in the nuclear medicine department of a hospital or large medical facility. Before receiving treatment, you will be informed about the regulations that govern the use of radiation, which are laid down by the Federal Government.

Following the treatment, you will be slightly radioactive for a number of days and your activities during that time are governed by the Nuclear Regulatory Commission, a branch of the United States Government.

You can understand why the Government might be concerned about the movement of radioactivity around the country, particularly in this post-9/11 world. However, you can rest assured that the amount of radiation you receive as treatment for hyperthyroidism is very small, and appears to be remarkably safe, with no significant increase in the risk of cancer or other serious health risks.

You will not represent a threat, either, to the health of others around you. Even so, you will receive instructions about avoiding places where you would come into contact with large groups of people, for example restaurants, movie theaters or bowling alleys. You should also avoid close or intimate contact with your partner and with young children or pregnant women for a few days after the treatment.

Radioactive iodine is never prescribed for pregnant women as it could damage the baby's thyroid gland. Women in the child-bearing age group are required to take a pregnancy test before receiving radioactive iodine treatment, even if they are sure they are not pregnant at the time. In addition, many specialists recommend that women avoid becoming pregnant for three or four months after treatment, to ensure that any effect of the radiation exposure is completely eliminated before a baby is conceived.

After treatment with radioactive iodine, patients whose thyroid has been severely overactive may be treated with beta-blockers or antithyroid drugs for a few weeks, to control the hyperthyroidism while the radioactive iodine takes effect. Blood tests after 8–12 weeks will usually confirm that the thyroid hormone levels have begun to fall below the normal range, at which time the endocrinologist will start treatment with thyroid hormone.

In about 5% of cases, a single dose of radioactive

Radioactive iodine treatment

Radioactive iodine is taken up by the thyroid gland, where it destroys part or all of the thyroid tissue, reducing the production of thyroid hormones.

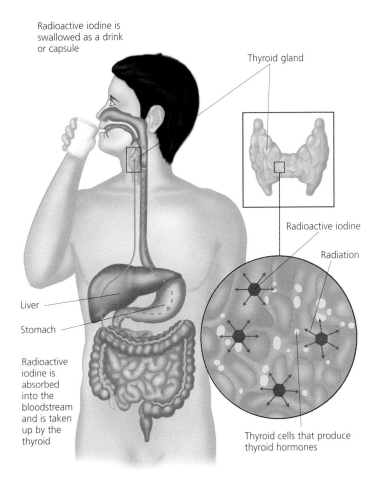

Radioactive iodine is swallowed as a drink or capsule

Thyroid gland

Radioactive iodine

Radiation

Liver

Stomach

Radioactive iodine is absorbed into the bloodstream and is taken up by the thyroid

Thyroid cells that produce thyroid hormones

Choosing which treatment is right for you after discussing each of the options with your endocrinologist

- The most popular treatment for hyperthyroidism in the US is radioactive iodine, because it is simple, effective, reliable, safe, and relatively inexpensive. However, not everyone is happy at the thought of using radioactivity for treatment, even if it is safe at the doses used for the treatment of hyperthyroidism. For them, either surgery or antithyroid drugs may be preferable.

- Sometimes Graves' disease can "burn itself out," which makes a second course of antithyroid drugs attractive for some patients, even if the condition comes back after a first course of these drugs. TMNG does not burn itself out, and one of the other treatments is generally preferred in these cases.

- Both surgery and radioactive iodine will usually cause the thyroid to become underactive. Patients who have been treated this way then need life-long treatment with thyroid hormone.

- Whatever kind of treatment you have for hyperthyroidism, you will need regular follow-ups, including a blood test taken at least once a year as part of your routine physical, to ensure that the TSH level remains normal.

iodine does not cure the hyperthyroidism, in which case you may need a second dose. That second dose is almost always effective.

Because the thyroid gland affected by TMNG doesn't take up as much iodine as a gland affected by Graves' disease, TMNG can be harder to treat with radioactive iodine, and the treatment is less likely to be effective, or to cause hypothyroidism. In some cases, the only effective treatment for TMNG might be surgery.

What you should know about radioactive iodine treatment

The main problem with radioactive iodine treatment is that it causes hypothyroidism. In fact, because hypothyroidism is generally easier to treat than hyperthyroidism, the development of an underactive thyroid is usually what the endocrinologist is aiming for.

Although some endocrinologists will try to come up with a dose of radioactive iodine that is "just right" and leaves enough of the gland functioning so that you do not need thyroid hormone treatment, this is rarely successful, and eventually most people become hypothyroid at some point after this treatment.

Even if your thyroid appears to return to normal initially after radioactive iodine treatment, it is essential that you have regular follow-up, at least annually, to detect hypothyroidism when it does finally develop. Once hypothyroidism has developed treatment is with thyroxine, most commonly in a dose of 100 to 150 micrograms once daily. Fortunately, there are no side effects with thyroxine if the appropriate dose is taken regularly.

Case history

At the age of 70, John Thornton was in generally good health. However, he recently noticed swelling of his ankles, worsening shortness of breath with exercise, and frequent strong heart beats, or palpitations.

One night, he woke up gasping for breath and coughing. His wife called 911 and he was hospitalized through the ER. The ER physician diagnosed heart failure as the cause of the fluid accumulation in John's legs and lungs.

He also found that John's pulse rate was rapid and irregular and an electrocardiogram (EKG) showed atrial fibrillation. John was treated with oxygen through a face-mask, an injection of the diuretic furosemide (Lasix™) to remove the excess fluid, and digoxin tablets to slow the heart rate. Because of the risk for patients with atrial fibrillation of developing blood clots, which might cause a stroke, he also received the blood thinner coumadin.

Because the attending cardiologist knew that atrial fibrillation could sometimes occur because of hyperthyroidism, she ordered lab work for thyroid tests. A low TSH and elevated thyroxine confirmed that John did indeed suffer from hyperthyroidism.

He was referred to an endocrinologist, who recommended starting PTU. After confirming that there had been no heart damage, John was able to leave the hospital within 24 hours. Within a month, his heart rhythm had returned entirely to normal, and his furosemide was stopped.

After stopping PTU for a few days, John was treated with radioactive iodine for what had been diagnosed as a toxic multinodular goiter (TMNG). Three months later, his thyroid tests showed the thyroid hormone levels falling and he was started on thyroxine tablets. All of his other medications, including the coumadin, were then withdrawn. His heart rate has remained stable since then, and he is back to his usual state of good health. He attends his internist once each year to check that his thyroid hormone levels are stable.

Case history

Anne Schwab was 32 when she first noticed hot flashes, sweating, and sensitivity to the heat. She feared that she might be suffering an early menopause, because her menstrual period was also becoming irregular and light.

When she began to lose weight and develop palpitations and a tremor, she feared something worse might be happening. She saw her family physician, who suspected hyperthyroidism, which he confirmed with lab tests.

Anne was referred to an endocrinologist in her home town, who arranged further testing with a thyroid uptake and scan. These studies confirmed a very overactive thyroid gland and a diagnosis of Graves' disease was made.

After a detailed discussion of the treatment options, Anne decided to avoid surgery, and preferred not to take radioactive iodine, because she had a two-year-old daughter at home. Instead, she chose a course of antithyroid drugs.

She started taking six tablets of PTU each day, and quickly noticed her symptoms settle. Although the tablets tasted bad, she put up with this side effect. Quickly, the dose of PTU was decreased, eventually to just one tablet daily, which she was able to take with her main meal of the day, with no side effects whatsoever.

Her thyroid hormone levels came under control, her

symptoms disappeared, and she felt normal. She took the PTU for 18 months, seeing her endocrinologist once every 3 months.

After the PTU was stopped, her thyroid hormone levels stayed normal and she now feels well three years later. She knows there is a chance that she could have further thyroid problems in the future, but all she needs is to have her thyroid checked every year by her family doctor.

Graves' disease and the eyes
What is happening in the eyes?
If you look carefully, most patients with Graves' disease have some changes to their eyes known as Graves' Eye Disease (GED). Ophthalmopathy, orbitopathy, exophthalmos, and proptosis are other terms used to describe these findings. Both eyes are usually affected, but often one is more severely affected than the other.

Usually the earliest sign of GED is retraction of the upper eyelid, which looks as if it has been pulled up, exposing more of the white of the eye and causing a staring appearance. Unlike most of the other changes, this feature may not improve after the hyperthyroidism is treated.

Many patients experience a dry, gritty sensation, which feels like dust or sand in the eyes. Excessive watering, sensitivity to bright lights, and constant blinking are other common features of the irritation to the eyes caused by GED.

The other features of GED are caused by a build-up of pressure behind the eyeball, which sits in a bony socket known as the orbit. The space between the eyeball and the back of the orbit contains the muscles that move the eye, the optic nerve which relays messages from the retina to the brain, and fatty tissue. GED causes an increase in the amount of fluid in this tissue behind the eyeball, causing swelling of the muscles and fat. As a result, the muscles may not be able to work efficiently, the normal movement of the eyes is affected, and double vision (diplopia), sometimes with a squint, may result. Often, the double vision occurs only when looking in a particular direction, or toward the end of the day when the patient is tired.

The increased pressure in the orbit pushes the eyeballs forward, producing a "bug-eyed" appearance, which is known technically as exophthalmos or proptosis. The increased pressure makes fluid drainage more difficult and the tissue around the eyes becomes

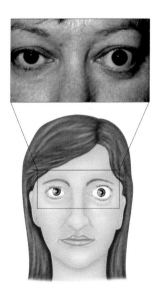

Most patients with Graves' disease will have some changes to their eyes, but most of the time these are very mild. Both eyes are usually affected but often one more than the other.

puffy and swollen, with prominent "bags" under (and over!) the eyes.

The forward movement of the eye makes it harder for the eyelids to close, allowing the eye to become dry and exposing it to irritation from dust, grit, wind, and sun. Often this problem is worst first thing in the morning, because the eye fails to close properly when you are asleep, and the front of the eye dries out overnight.

In severe cases, exposure of the outer lining of the eye (the cornea) can cause damage to the eye, while high pressure at the back of the eye can compress the optic nerve, causing partial or total loss of vision. Fortunately, these serious problems are rare, and can usually be prevented or corrected with appropriate treatment.

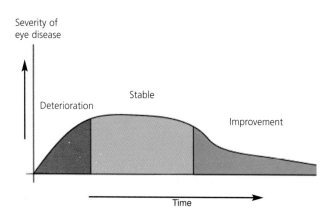

Thyroid-related eye disease usually has three phases, each of variable duration. After an initial deterioration the condition should stabilize over a period of two to three years. Thereafter relatively minor surgery should correct any double vision and improve the cosmetic appearance of the eyes.

There are three phases to GED:

- the initial development and worsening of symptoms,
- followed by stabilization
- followed by some improvement

Most people with Graves' disease have only very mild changes in the eyes, which may not even be noticeable, except to a specialist endocrinologist or ophthalmologist. For these people, treatment is usually not needed, the problem stabilizes on its own, and any visible symptoms fade away in a few months. However, complete disappearance of GED is rare and, even if you feel that your eyes are back to normal, there will probably be subtle abnormalities evident to a specialist.

GED is really a separate autoimmune condition, which frequently coexists with Graves' disease, and is not really a complication of the thyroid disease itself. It is important to remember that treatment of the thyroid may not help the eyes, and changes in the eyes may not tell you anything about whether the thyroid has been properly treated. Sometimes, GED can occur long before the thyroid gland becomes overactive. In other cases, GED develops only long after the thyroid gland has been successfully treated. In most cases, however, GED and hyperthyroidism come on around the same time and are diagnosed together.

Treatment
Treatment of GED is not as straightforward as treatment of hyperthyroidism. Smoking makes GED worse, so quitting smoking is an important part of the treatment. Avoiding secondhand smoke is also worthwhile. Treatment of hyperthyroidism and

hypothyroidism may also help GED. So keeping the thyroid hormone levels perfect is important.

There is some concern that radioactive iodine treatment for hyperthyroidism could make GED worse, and some endocrinologists will avoid this treatment for patients with bad GED. However, a course of steroids (such as prednisone) taken for a few weeks after radioactive iodine treatment can prevent any worsening of the eyes, and in the long term, radioactive iodine seems to be just as safe as surgery or antithyroid drugs as far as the eyes are concerned.

Artificial tears, available over the counter in most drug stores, can help to ease symptoms of dry eyes

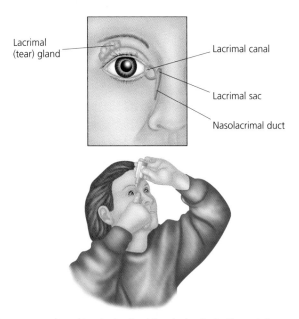

Tears are produced by the lacrimal (tear) glands. In Graves' disease they may not work as well as normal. If you have dry eyes artificial tears may help relieve the discomfort.

and grittiness, though they need to be used frequently. They may also help relieve watery eyes, which are triggered by dryness and irritation. Sunglasses can help with light sensitivity. Cool compresses over the eyes may also relieve some of the symptoms.

Double vision, blurred vision, and other worrisome symptoms should be assessed by an ophthalmologist experienced in management of GED. Correction of double vision can sometimes be achieved by special prism lenses fitted to eyeglasses, or by blocking the vision from one of the eyes by use of a patch.

High pressure behind the eye can be relieved by courses of steroids (prednisone), though often very high doses are required. Radiotherapy (X-ray treatment) to the eye has been used on patients with severe GED, though it is not clear just how useful this approach really is.

When the pressure behind the eye threatens to cause blindness, surgery to relieve the pressure on the optic nerve may be necessary. This surgery, which should be carried out by a highly experienced ophthalmologist, involves removing part of the bone of the orbit to relieve the pressure behind the eye. Although it is usually very successful, this type of surgery is only used in severe GED. Typically, a second surgery is needed later to correct the double vision that the first surgery is likely to cause.

Fortunately, most people with Graves' disease find that their eye problems are mild, do not require anything other than some eye-drops to relieve dryness, and settle down within a few months to a year or two. Minor surgery can sometimes be used to correct any "staring" look, or bags under the eyes that remain once the GED has stabilized.

Less common causes of hyperthyroidism

- Mild hyperthyroidism, lasting for a few weeks, may occur after a viral infection. Sometimes the viral infection causes quite severe pain and tenderness over the thyroid gland, as well as symptoms of a flu-like illness. This condition is known as "viral thyroiditis" or "de Quervain's thyroiditis." In other cases, there is no thyroid pain or tenderness, and only the hyperthyroidism occurs, a condition known as "silent thyroiditis." In either case, the hyperthyroidism rarely needs any treatment other than a beta-blocker, such as propranolol. The pain of viral thyroiditis may respond to anti-inflammatory drugs, or to high doses of steroids (prednisone). The hyperthyroidism usually lasts a few weeks, and is followed by an equally short-lived period of hypothyroidism. Most patients make a full recovery.

- Amiodarone is a drug used by cardiologists to treat an abnormal heart rhythm. It contains a very large amount of iodine; in fact, one 200mg tablet of amiodarone contains 500 times the recommended daily allowance of iodine! Iodine in this very large amount can sometimes trigger thyroid problems, including hypothyroidism or hyperthyroidism. Most cardiologists recommend regular testing of the thyroid during treatment with amiodarone.

- The combination of a low TSH and normal T_3 and T_4 levels in the blood is known as subclinical hyperthyroidism, because most patients have few, if any, symptoms. This abnormality is usually detected during a routine thyroid test. It is the mildest form of thyroid overactivity and treatment is often recommended, even if you feel perfectly well, to try to prevent osteoporosis or atrial fibrillation, and to avoid true hyperthyroidism developing in the future.

KEY POINTS

- Around 75% of cases of hyperthyroidism are caused by Graves' disease

- Many people with Graves' disease have inherited a tendency to develop it, but other factors seem to trigger the condition

- The people most likely to develop Graves' disease are women between the ages of 30 and 50, with a family history of thyroid problems or other inflammatory diseases. However, other people can also be affected

- Antithyroid drugs, surgery, and radioactive iodine are all effective in treating Graves' disease, but there is no one treatment that is right for everyone, and none of these treatments is perfect

- Your endocrinologist will want to discuss the treatment options with you before making the final decision on which approach is best for you

- Radioactive iodine is the most popular treatment in the US for patients with hyperthyroidism. It is generally safe, simple, effective, and relatively inexpensive

- Agranulocytosis is a rare side effect of antithyroid drugs. It is a medical emergency and you must contact your physician or hospital immediately to be assessed the same day

■ Most people with Graves' disease will have changes in the eyes, but in most cases, these problems are mild. More serious symptoms can be treated and usually settle in time

■ After treatment for hyperthyroidism, you need regular follow-up to make sure that your thyroid hormone levels remain normal

Underactive thyroid (hypothyroidism)

What is an underactive thyroid?

An underactive thyroid (hypothyroidism) occurs when the thyroid gland stops producing enough of the thyroid hormones, T_3 and T_4. The most common form seen in the US is known as "Hashimoto's disease," which affects between 1 and 5 percent of the population, especially women over the age of 50, though younger women and men may also be affected.

Hashimoto's disease

This condition is the result of an immune system attack on the thyroid, which injures, damages, weakens, and ultimately destroys the thyroid gland. In doing so, the thyroid commonly enlarges, developing a goiter, as a result both of the inflammation and an effort by the thyroid to continue to do its job effectively.

Typically, Hashimoto's disease begins in early adult life, progressing gradually over many years. During this time, the thyroid gland continues to produce thyroid hormone normally, and in most cases the patient experiences no symptoms whatsoever, except, perhaps the development of a goiter.

Ultimately, however, the gland weakens to the point that it can no longer make enough thyroid hormone for the body's needs. At that point, the patient develops progressive symptoms of hypothyroidism.

Atrophic hypothyroidism (Ord's disease)

A second form of hypothyroidism is "atrophic hypothyroidism," otherwise known as Ord's disease, which is also caused by an immune system attack on the gland. In this case, the thyroid gland shrinks as its cells are destroyed by the immune system, so that no goiter is formed.

Many patients with this condition are actually told they have Hashimoto's disease. However, because the treatment of Hashimoto's disease and atrophic hypothyroidism are the same, this misdiagnosis is probably not all that important for most patients. Poor Dr. Ord has lost out in history to his more famous colleague, Dr. Hashimoto!

The role of the immune system

Like Graves' disease, discussed previously on page 10, both major types of hypothyroidism are caused by the immune system. Once again, these conditions are associated with the other "autoimmune diseases" shown in the box on page 53.

Although having hypothyroidism makes you somewhat more likely to develop one or more of these conditions, remember that the risk is still small, and most people with a thyroid problem will never experience any of these other conditions.

Autoimmune diseases associated with hypothyroidism

- Pernicious anemia, causing vitamin B_{12} deficiency, for which regular injections of vitamin B_{12} are necessary to maintain a normal blood count

- Diabetes mellitus requiring treatment with insulin

- Addison's disease: the adrenal glands, which sit above the kidneys, weaken and stop producing cortisol and aldosterone, hormones that are essential for life but which, fortunately, can be taken as tablets

- Premature ovarian failure which causes loss of periods, infertility, and an early menopause

- Underactivity of the parathyroid glands, which lie behind the thyroid, leading to a low level of calcium in the blood. This can be treated with vitamin D capsules

- Vitiligo, a skin disease in which there are areas of loss of pigment, giving a "piebald" appearance

What is the pattern of development?

Hypothyroidism usually develops slowly over many months, so it is common for the symptoms to go unnoticed, particularly in older people, who may simply put them down to aging. Nowadays, more and more physicians send lab work for thyroid testing as part of a routine physical exam, at least in patients at particular risk for developing thyroid disease. As a result, more patients are being detected at a very early stage, often well before any symptoms have developed. This is good, of course, because it allows treatment to be started early, and symptoms can be avoided.

Unfortunately, it can sometimes have the effect of encouraging both patients and physicians to be unrealistic about what thyroid hormone replacement might do. In most cases, thyroid hormone treatment at a very early stage of hypothyroidism will not produce any real improvement in the patient's health and will not make them feel any better. The purpose of treatment in these early cases is simply to prevent new symptoms from developing.

Despite the availability of early testing, diagnosis may still be delayed in some patients and they will go on to develop full-blown hypothyroidism, known in its advanced state as "myxedema." In those cases, all or most of the symptoms listed below are likely to be present.

Of course, in milder cases, diagnosed earlier, the extent and the severity of these symptoms is likely to be much less. You will notice, as well, that many of these symptoms are quite vague and non-specific. It is important for a physician trying to diagnose a thyroid problem to take into account both the pattern and the severity of the symptoms, as well as how those symptoms fit together, and to avoid the temptation of blaming every symptom on the thyroid!

Symptoms of hypothyroidism
Weight gain
Weight gain from hypothyroidism tends to come on slowly and progressively, despite efforts at diet and exercise. On average, patients with hypothyroidism have gained between 10 and 20 pounds by the time the diagnosis is made.

It is very unusual to gain more weight than this, except in severe myxedema, when weight gain of up to 30 or 40 pounds may rarely be seen. Weight gain greater than these amounts, is hardly ever caused by the thyroid, and other causes should be considered.

Sensitivity to the cold
You'll feel the cold badly, want to wear extra layers of clothing, turn up the heat even in summer, or sit close to the fire. You might also experience muscle stiffness and cramping when you move suddenly, especially when it's cold.

Fatigue, tiredness, and mental problems
Tiredness, sleepiness, and slowing down intellectually are common features of hypothyroidism. Your reactions tend to become slower, so some patients may feel unsafe driving or operating dangerous machinery. Older patients may be suspected to be suffering from Alzheimer's disease, while others might experience depression or mood swings.

Speech
Your voice becomes slow and husky and speech is often slurred. This tends to occur only in quite severe hypothyroidism.

Heart
In contrast to a person with an overactive thyroid gland, your pulse rate is slow, at around 60 beats per minute. You may have high blood pressure and an elderly patient with severe long-standing hypothyroidism is at risk of heart failure. Angina may also be the first symptom of hypothyroidism.

Bowel movements
You will tend to develop constipation.

Menstruation
Women before menopause may notice heavier than normal periods (menorrhagia).

Skin and hair
Your skin is likely to be coarse, dry, and flaky. It tends to be pale and the eyelids, hands, and feet become puffy. Some people may find that their skin becomes yellowish, while prominent blood vessels in the cheeks may add a purple tinge.

Some people develop vitiligo, a skin condition in which areas of the skin lose their pigment. The hair becomes dry and brittle and the outer part of the eyebrows may be lost.

Nervous system
In severe cases of hypothyroidism, you may become hard of hearing, have trouble with your balance, or develop tingling in the fingers, suggesting carpal tunnel syndrome.

Confirming the diagnosis
Blood test
In most cases, a simple blood test is sufficient to confirm a diagnosis of hypothyroidism. The most accurate single test is the TSH level, which can be performed accurately by most labs. The finding of a high TSH level strongly suggests that the thyroid is weakened, and that hypothyroidism is present.

The high TSH tells the physician that the body is calling on the thyroid to work harder, a sign that there is not enough thyroid hormone in the circulation. Measurement of the T_4 and T_3 levels can also help to confirm this.

Measurement of the thyroid antibody levels in the blood (Thyroid Peroxidase Antibodies (TPO), or Thyroglobulin antibodies (Tg)) can help confirm that the problem is Hashimoto's disease or Ord's disease.

Interpreting test results
No symptoms, elevated TSH
In a person with no symptoms, in whom a TSH is found to be slightly high, it is worth remembering that each of us will occasionally develop a high TSH temporarily, especially following a viral or other illness, as the body is recovering. In those cases, it is worth waiting a few weeks and repeating the tests, rather than rushing in with a treatment which needs to be taken for the patient's whole life!

Symptoms, normal TSH
An equally common situation, though much more confusing, is a patient who has symptoms of an underactive thyroid, but in whom the TSH turns out to be normal. There are three possible reasons for this situation.

First, the TSH might be "wrong." Although it is very unusual, it is possible for a lab to get the test wrong, for a sample to be mixed up with someone else's, or for some other technical problem to interfere with the results. Under those conditions, repeating the lab work, while also measuring the T_4 and T_3 levels, can help to point the physician in the right direction.

The second possibility is that the TSH measurement is right, but that the body simply cannot make enough

TSH. Most of these very rare cases turn out to be caused by a problem with the pituitary gland, which requires evaluation and treatment by an endocrinologist. Measurement of the T_4 and T_3 levels will usually point the physician in the right direction in these cases too.

The third cause of hypothyroid symptoms with a normal level of TSH occurs because the hypothyroid symptoms are not very specific, and can often be caused by some other condition, which mimics hypothyroidism. This condition is discussed in more detail in a later chapter of this book.

Finding the correct cause of symptoms

Many of us experience weight gain, despite trying to be sensible with our diet. Many more of us experience fatigue and tiredness, often because of sleep disturbance, or worrying too much about our job, finances, children, or parents.

Sometimes, disease of other types causes symptoms that overlap with those of hypothyroidism. A more detailed discussion of "hypothyroidism with normal thyroid tests" begins on page 134.

This issue becomes a particular problem for a patient who has a mild thyroid problem and who is then disappointed when treatment of the thyroid fails to cure the symptoms. It is tempting for the physician and the patient simply to continue to adjust the dose of thyroid hormone, while failing to realize that the problem may actually lie elsewhere.

All too often it seems, the physician is focused on the fact that the thyroid tests are now "normal," while the patient is frustrated that the symptoms are no better! As usual in medicine, both patient and physician need to be on the same page. One purpose of this book is to make sure that you and your physician can at least speak the same language.

Treatment of hypothyroidism

Hypothyroidism is usually treated with pure thyroxine (T_4, or levothyroxine), taken once daily by mouth. Almost always, treatment with thyroxine, once started, needs to be taken lifelong.

Several different brands of thyroxine are sold, and

Treatment for an underactive thyroid gland (hypothyroidism)

Before
The thyroid gland produces inadequate amounts of thyroid hormones

After
Thyroxine taken by mouth supplements the low thyroid hormones and is converted by the body to the active hormone T_3

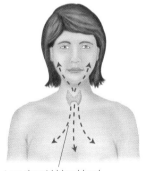

Low thyroid blood level

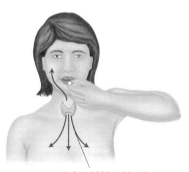

Normal thyroid blood level

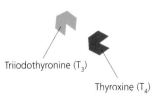

Triiodothyronine (T_3)

Thyroxine (T_4)

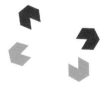

a generic version is also available. All require a prescription. Brand names include Synthroid™, Levothroid™, Levoxyl™, Unithroid™, and Euthyrox™. The generic form is sold under the name Levothyroxine.

Each of the brands—and the generic medication— are available in a wide variety of strengths, including tablets containing 25, 50, 75, 88, 100, 112, 125, 137, 150, 175, 200, 250, and 300 micrograms (mcg).

Most adult patients eventually need between 100 and 150 mcg daily. It is common to start treatment at a low dose and to increase the dose gradually, blood tests being performed about 2–3 months after starting a new dose, and the dose adjusted to reach the target level of TSH and thyroid hormones.

The goal is usually to achieve a normal, stable level of TSH and thyroid hormones in the blood. Once the ideal dose has been found, the frequency of testing can gradually be extended, eventually to once-a-year testing, because the need for thyroid hormone tends to be stable throughout life, varying only slightly with age.

Do different varieties of thyroxine have the same effect?

According to the Food and Drug Administration (FDA), most of the brands of thyroid hormone, and the generic levothyroxine, are "bioequivalent," meaning that they have the same biological effects, and can be used interchangeably.

However, most endocrinologists, with far more knowledge and experience of thyroid disease than the FDA, do not agree with this position, because we see some patients who experience significant changes in

TSH and thyroid hormone levels when they are switched from one brand to another.

This is particularly true of patients with thyroid cancer, for whom the ideal range of TSH is much narrower than patients with hypothyroidism, but it applies to some patients with hypothyroidism too.

If your insurer, pharmacist, or physician require you to switch between brands, or between a brand name and the generic, you should have your TSH rechecked 2–3 months later to make sure the levels remain stable.

Most patients find that their symptoms of hypothyroidism start to improve within a week or two of starting treatment with thyrosine, but a full recovery can take 3–6 months, or even longer, particularly for patients with long-standing or severe hypothyroidism. Recovery from symptoms can also take longer for patients who had hyperthyroidism, but who develop hypothyroidism after treatment of the overactive thyroid.

For most patients, getting the TSH into the normal range causes all of the symptoms of hypothyroidism to disappear, with a return to normal health.

A few patients are very sensitive to the effects of thyroxine and feel better when the TSH level is at, or close to, the upper or the lower ends of the normal range.

If your symptoms of hypothyroidism persist, or if you develop symptoms of hyperthyroidism while taking thyroxine, you and your physician can adjust the dose further, even when your TSH level is "normal," to try to give you the maximum benefit. For most patients, this optimal level comes when the TSH lies in the lowest third of the normal range (a TSH of 0.5–2.0 mU/L for most labs).

Importance of stability

Almost as important as the level of TSH and thyroid hormone in the blood is having a stable level. Frequent, major changes in thyroid hormone dose should be avoided if possible. Unstable levels of thyroid hormone are often caused by failing to take the medicine reliably, or by taking it in the wrong way.

Ideally, thyroid hormone should be taken first thing in the morning, on an empty stomach, 45–60 minutes before food. Alternatively, it can be taken three or four hours after a meal, once the stomach has emptied.

What can interfere with thyroid hormone absorption?

Many different medicines, including vitamins, minerals, and various supplements, can interfere with thyroid hormone absorption, so thyroid hormone should be taken alone, no other medication being taken at the same time. This is particularly important in the case of iron and calcium supplements, or multivitamins that contain these elements.

Some drugs can interfere with thyroid hormone metabolism. A partial list of these drugs is given on page 67. If your doctor is giving you a new prescription, stopping a previous prescription, or changing the dose of any of these drugs, make sure she or he is aware that you are taking thyroid hormone, and ask whether the change might interfere with the thyroid hormone dose. If in doubt, make sure that you have your thyroid hormone levels checked after 2–3 months to ensure they are stable.

Remembering to take any medication every day is a struggle for all of us, and thyroid hormone is no exception. Once in a while, it is worth double-checking to make sure that you are not missing out any of your medication accidentally. To do this, simply count the number of tablets in the bottle once a week for a few weeks, and make sure that you have really taken seven tablets each week. It is amazing how often someone will find that—completely unknowingly—they missed out a dose or two, or took an extra dose, without even being aware of it. This can lead to a very significant change in the dose of thyroid hormone being received, and can dramatically affect the stability of your thyroid hormone levels.

Case history

Jean Tollefson was 18 years old, a high school senior, who felt she was struggling to keep up in her classes. She was tired, cold, and having a hard time keeping her weight down. She contracted Type 1 diabetes at age 11, and was taking three injections of insulin each day, but noticed she was having a harder time controlling her blood sugars recently. She had developed a low blood sugar more frequently in the last few weeks, and on one occasion, she had almost lost consciousness in class due to hypoglycemia.

It was her aunt, visiting from California, who recognized the change in Jean's appearance since her last visit the previous year. She herself had developed an underactive thyroid gland 10 years earlier and suggested to Jean that she have a blood test.

The blood test was positive, showing a very high level of TSH and low level of T_4, with positive antibodies in the blood. Because of the family history, her internist recommended family screening and her mom was also found to have an underactive thyroid, though at an early stage. Jean—and her mom— are now taking thyroxine, like her aunt.

Jean is feeling fine and will be ready to start college in the fall. Her diabetes control is back to normal with less hypoglycemia, and her weight is down to its normal level, though it took six to eight months—and a lot of hard work with diet and exercise—to get there.

Special situations
Angina

Treatment with thyroxine can worsen angina (heart pain caused by narrowed blood vessels—coronary artery disease). If you suffer from angina, your doctor may use a lower dose of thyroxine than usual to start treatment of hypothyroidism, and may choose to increase the dose more slowly and more cautiously than usual.

Sometimes, coronary artery bypass grafting (CABG) or angioplasty (opening a narrowed blood vessel with a balloon) may be necessary before thyroxine treatment can be tolerated, though this is unusual.

Temporary hypothyroidism

Treatment with thyroxine is usually needed lifelong. However, if you develop hypothyroidism in the first three to four months after surgery or radioactive iodine treatment for Graves' disease, it can be short-lived, lasting only a few weeks, and you may not need any treatment. The same is true for hypothyroidism caused by viral thyroiditis (page 48), or triggered by pregnancy (page 77).

Mild (subclinical) hypothyroidism

A mildly elevated TSH (between 5 and 10 mU/L) can often be seen with normal levels of T_4 and T_3 in people with no symptoms of thyroid disease. Some of these

The process of atherosclerosis

Atherosclerosis, atheroma, and hardening of the arteries are all the same thing—the process leading to the blockage or weakening of arteries.

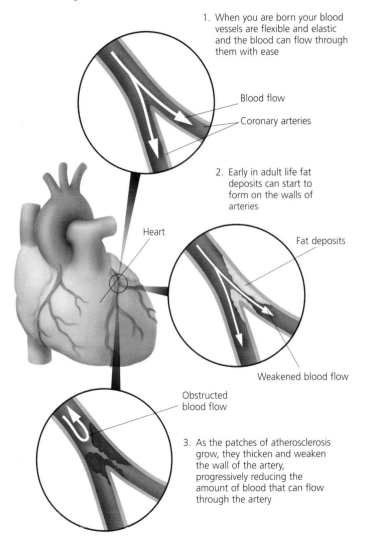

1. When you are born your blood vessels are flexible and elastic and the blood can flow through them with ease

Blood flow

Coronary arteries

2. Early in adult life fat deposits can start to form on the walls of arteries

Fat deposits

Heart

Weakened blood flow

Obstructed blood flow

3. As the patches of atherosclerosis grow, they thicken and weaken the wall of the artery, progressively reducing the amount of blood that can flow through the artery

people will go on to develop true hypothyroidism and require treatment with thyroxine.

However, some patients remain stable for many years and in others, the TSH level returns to normal. For such sufferers, treatment with thyroxine may not be necessary. However, if the TSH is rising on sequential tests, and is above 10–12 mU/L, if there is a family history of thyroid disease, if there are thyroid antibodies in the blood, or if the patient has any symptoms that might hint at hypothyroidism, it is common practice nowadays to go ahead and treat with thyroxine.

There is truth to the adage that "an ounce of prevention is worth a pound of cure." Having said that, some patients and their physicians prefer to avoid unnecessary treatment and simply monitor the situation with regular blood tests.

Hypothyroidism caused by drugs

Lithium is a drug used to treat some forms of manic depression and other psychiatric problems that lead to unstable mood. Lithium can cause both a goiter and hypothyroidism. If the lithium is felt to be necessary to keep the mood disorder under control, treatment with thyroxine will be needed to overcome the effects of lithium on the thyroid.

As noted on page 48, Amiodarone, which is used to treat some heart rhythm problems, can cause either hyperthyroidism or hypothyroidism, and anyone taking Amiodarone will need to have thyroid blood tests from time to time.

Changes to your usual dose of thyroxine

The dose of thyroxine will probably need to be increased during pregnancy (see pages 77–78).

Some commonly used drugs that may increase the need for thyroxine

Drug	Use
Carbamazepine (Tegretol™)	Control of epilepsy
Sertraline (Zoloft™)	Antidepressant
Ferrous sulphate (Iron supplement)	Treatment of anemia
estrogen	Contraception, menopausal symptoms
Calcium	Osteoporosis prevention
Multivitamin	General health

Poor absorption of thyroxine from the stomach is uncommon, but can occur in untreated celiac disease. Similarly, if you start taking medication that reduces the absorption of thyroxine or speeds up its metabolism, the dose of thyroxine may need to be changed.

Typically, your physician will be guided by the level of TSH in the blood, which is a very reliable indicator of your body's need for thyroid hormone.

Treatment with T$_3$ (Cytomel™, Liothyronine™) and "Natural" thyroid hormone (Armour thyroid™)

Most patients with hypothyroidism make a full recovery after starting treatment with thyroxine, and have no symptoms, while taking an appropriate dose of the medication, adjusted according to their TSH level.

Others, however, do not make such a good recovery and continue to experience hypothyroid symptoms, even though their TSH is "normal." Some patients feel better if they take some extra thyroxine, even though this causes a low TSH level. This leads their physician to be concerned about the effect of hyperthyroidism on the risk of osteoporosis or heart rhythm problems (atrial fibrillation). This can lead to a conflict in which the physician wants to keep the dose of thyroxine low, while the patient pushes for a higher dose. Not surprisingly, disagreements of this type can damage the patient's trust in his or her physician.

Before letting this disagreement develop into a full-blown argument, it is worth remembering what was said on page 56 ("Confirming the diagnosis") about the fact that many of the symptoms of hypothyroidism resemble the symptoms of many other conditions.

Before assuming that the problem "must" be caused by the thyroid, it is worth a very careful evaluation to exclude the possibility that some other problem is causing the symptoms, as these would not respond to thyroxine treatment. Sometimes, referral to an endocrinologist or other specialist is necessary before reaching a conclusion. A discussion of this issue is included starting on page 134 ("Hypothyroidism with normal blood tests").

Treatment of persistent hypothyroid symptoms

Despite all of these evaluations, a small number of patients with hypothyroidism suffer persistent hypothyroid symptoms, despite what should be an adequate dose of thyroid hormone. For these patients, there are three possible approaches that can sometimes be useful.

First approach

The simplest approach is merely to increase the dose of thyroxine (T_4), until the patient feels better, accepting that the TSH will fall and the blood tests might suggest hyperthyroidism.

There are, of course, some risks to this approach, including risks to the bones (osteoporosis) and the heart. Some patients consider these risks worth taking, if they make them feel sufficiently better, but not all doctors will be willing or comfortable in allowing this approach, and certainly a full discussion of the risks, and careful monitoring for any complications, is essential if this path is followed.

Second approach

The second approach, which may not actually be any safer, however, is to use a combination of thyroxine with a small dose of T_3, available commercially as Cytomel™ or Liothyronine™. Typically, the dose of thyroxine will be reduced somewhat (say 125mcg down to 100mcg), with the T_3 added in a dose of 5mcg twice daily.

Although it is often argued that this T_3 supplement is "more physiological" than T_4 treatment alone, there is a real drawback, because all of the T_3 drugs available have a short duration of action, and therefore have to be taken in small doses several times each day.

Even so, this approach seems to be helpful for a small number of patients who cannot find relief for their symptoms in any other way. Typically, the physician will try to find the combination of T_4 and T_3 that keeps the TSH normal (usually toward the low end of the normal range), and both the T_4 and T_3 toward the high end of their normal ranges.

The main drawbacks of this approach are that it is harder to monitor and adjust, and that it leaves the patient prone to swings in the T_3 level, in particular, which can leave them feeling "groggy" as the T_3 dose wears off.

Third approach

The third approach is to go back to the original form of thyroid hormone replacement, and use a thyroid extract derived from animal thyroid tissue. This "natural" form of thyroid hormone replacement was used effectively to treat hypothyroidism for many years, before levothyroxine became available. It suffers from some variability in the strength, between batches, and tends to contain rather too much T_3 compared to T_4, so that it probably isn't really "natural" for a human being.

Even so, this approach is a reasonable and safe one for patients who feel better on this form of thyroid hormone replacement. Adjustment of the dose is performed in the usual way, using the level of TSH in the blood to get the dose right. Monitoring often has to be more intense, because of the variability in the strength of these tablets.

KEY POINTS

- Hypothyroidism usually comes on slowly and the symptoms are likely to be vague at first

- The diagnosis is usually straightforward, with a simple blood test confirming hypothyroidism

- Thyroid hormone replacement is the appropriate treatment, which you will probably need to take for the rest of your life

- Patients with coronary artery disease may need to start thyroxine at a lower dose and increase the dose slowly, to avoid worsening their heart condition

- If the thyroid blood test is only slightly abnormal, you may either be monitored, or be given thyroxine to prevent symptoms in the future

- Treatment with thyroid hormone requires lifelong monitoring, typically once a year

Thyroid disease and pregnancy

Will thyroid disease stop me becoming pregnant?

Women with a thyroid problem will almost always be able to become pregnant, so long as the thyroid is treated properly beforehand. During pregnancy, treatment of a thyroid problem may have to be adjusted, and more intensive monitoring is often recommended.

Thyroid disease may occur for the first time during or after a pregnancy, perhaps because the thyroid has to work much harder during a pregnancy than at other times. Thyroid problems in the mother can affect the health and development of the baby, so careful attention to the thyroid problem is important.

Graves' disease and pregnancy

Hyperthyroidism occurring during pregnancy is rare, but when it happens, it is almost always caused by Graves' disease. The symptoms of hyperthyroidism are the same as they would be in someone who is not pregnant, but in addition, nausea and vomiting are frequent symptoms of hyperthyroidism in pregnancy.

These symptoms are often blamed on morning sickness, while heat intolerance and rapid heartbeat are attributed to the hormonal changes of pregnancy. Emotional changes may be blamed on the pregnancy rather than attributed to the thyroid.

Although the blood tests that are used to diagnose thyroid problems are still accurate during a pregnancy, changes in a woman's hormone levels can make those thyroid tests harder to interpret accurately. In addition, to avoid exposing the baby to any radiation, the scans and uptake measurement often used to evaluate thyroid problems (see page 24) cannot be performed during pregnancy, which makes the diagnosis a little more difficult. Close cooperation between your obstetrician and an endocrinologist is the best way to ensure that these problems do not prevent accurate diagnosis.

During pregnancy, Graves' disease cannot be treated with radioactive iodine, because the radiation would destroy the baby's thyroid, and might also injure the baby in other ways. As a result, the choice of treatment lies between antithyroid drugs and surgery.

Surgery for Graves' disease is not often used during pregnancy, but can be performed during the middle of the pregnancy—the second trimester (between about 16 and 26 weeks). Earlier than this, there is a concern about the effect of the anesthetic on the health of the baby; later on, there is an increased risk of triggering premature labor.

Much more commonly, the choice is made to use antithyroid drugs (PTU or MMZ) to control the hyperthyroidism. This is both effective for the mother

The placenta

The fetus depends on the mother for oxygen and nutrients. The placenta allows the exchange of oxygen and nourishment between the mother and the fetus.

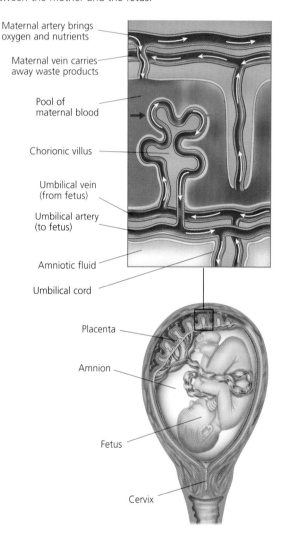

Maternal artery brings oxygen and nutrients

Maternal vein carries away waste products

Pool of maternal blood

Chorionic villus

Umbilical vein (from fetus)

Umbilical artery (to fetus)

Amniotic fluid

Umbilical cord

Placenta

Amnion

Fetus

Cervix

and safe for the baby. The thyroid-stimulating antibody responsible for the hyperthyroidism of Graves' disease actually crosses the placenta and causes the baby to have an overactive thyroid gland too. Fortunately, the antithyroid drugs also cross the placenta and good control of hyperthyroidism in the mother will ensure that the baby is not harmed.

If the hyperthyroidism is not adequately treated, a miscarriage can result, while overtreatment with antithyroid drugs may lead to a goiter in the baby. For these reasons, it is important that the patient is prescribed the lowest dose of PTU possible to keep the thyroid hormone levels normal. Usually, these levels are checked every four to six weeks throughout the pregnancy. The carbimazole is then stopped four weeks before the baby's due date, to make sure that baby is not hypothyroid at such a crucial time in its development.

If hyperthyroidism recurs in the mother after the baby is born, and if she is breast-feeding at the time, she can again be treated with PTU, though MMZ is generally avoided because it is secreted in the milk to a greater extent, and might affect the baby.

PTU is very safe when used in pregnancy in low doses. Although there is some concern about a rare disease in the newborn baby, called *aplasia cutis,* in which there is a defect in the skin covering a small part of the scalp, this risk is actually very small and the problem can be treated quite easily if it does happen.

Hyperthyroidism in the newborn (neonatal thyrotoxicosis)

In most women with Graves' disease during pregnancy, the thyroid-stimulating antibody disappears or its level in the blood becomes very low, especially toward the end of the pregnancy. In a few women, however, the level remains high and, as blood from the mother is exchanged with that of the fetus until the moment of birth, these high levels are also present in the blood of the newborn.

In these cases, the newborn baby can suffer from hyperthyroidism. Hyperthyroidism in the newborn, if detected early, is quite easily treated and lasts only two to three weeks until the antibody from the mother is broken down and deactivated.

Very occasionally, mothers who have been treated successfully for Graves' disease in the past continue to produce thyroid-stimulating antibody and their babies are at risk of developing neonatal hyperthyroidism. Measurement of the TSH-receptor antibody (TRAb) level can help to identify these few women, whose babies can then be screened at birth.

Case history

Rebecca Sellner and her husband had been trying to have a second child for three years without success. Rebecca had conceived twice, but on each occasion had miscarried at about ten weeks. She felt and looked well and, although she had lost a few pounds in weight, she put this down to her busy life, as a full-time secretary, looking after an active five-year-old son, and keeping up with all her homemaking tasks.

Finally, worried that she might never be able to have another baby, she attended a fertility specialist's clinic, which recommended she be tested for thyroid hormone levels. She knew that one of her cousins had recently been diagnosed with an underactive thyroid, but was surprised to learn that the lab work showed she had mild hyperthyroidism, which was confirmed as Graves' disease by the endocrinologist. Treatment was recommended with radioactive iodine, but instead, Rebecca chose PTU. Quickly her thyroid hormone levels became normal, and after five months of treatment, Rebecca became pregnant.

She was seen by her endocrinologist every six weeks during the pregnancy and the PTU was stopped four weeks before the expected date of delivery. She gave birth to a healthy girl whose heel-prick blood test was normal, with no evidence of thyroid problems. Rebecca breast-fed her daughter but, after four months, developed hyperthyroidism again. She decided to restart propylthiouracil and continue breast-feeding, rather than stop breast-feeding and take radioactive iodine. She is considering whether surgery would be right for her, if the thyroid flares up again in the future, but won't make that decision until she has to.

Hypothyroidism and pregnancy

Most women with hypothyroidism are already taking thyroxine when they become pregnant. Although mild hypothyroidism may not affect fertility, women with severe hypothyroidism are less likely to become pregnant. If they do become pregnant, spontaneous miscarriage is very likely.

The dose of thyroxine often has to be increased during pregnancy. Thyroid hormone is very important to the developing baby, especially in the first few weeks of a pregnancy. As a result, women with an underactive thyroid who are planning to become pregnant should be tested before conception, and should have their dose of thyroid hormone made as close to perfect as possible.

During those first few weeks of the pregnancy, the goal of treatment should be to keep the TSH level toward the low end of the normal range—in other words, keeping the thyroid hormone levels a little higher than average.

Recent research shows that the increase is most important to the fetus in early pregnancy. Some endocrinologists suggest that, as soon as you know that you are pregnant, you should increase your dose of thyroxine by 25 mcg daily, and have a blood test. You should certainly have your blood monitored throughout the pregnancy, ideally every 6 to 8 weeks. The average woman needs an increase of between 30 and 50 percent above their baseline dose. Once the baby is delivered, you can return to the dose you were taking before pregnancy.

Although the baby's thyroid gland develops independently of the mother and starts making thyroid hormones after about 12 weeks, a recent study has shown that hypothyroidism affecting the mother, which is either unrecognized or inadequately treated, can cause the baby's IQ to be lower than it should be. As a result, making sure you take your thyroid hormone regularly, reliably, and appropriately, and that your physician keeps the dose as near perfect as possible, is important throughout a pregnancy.

It probably also makes sense for women—at least those with a family history of thyroid disease—to have their thyroid checked when planning a pregnancy, however, this is not yet a recommendation that is accepted by all obstetricians, because of the cost.

Hypothyroidism in the newborn (congenital hypothyroidism)

About 1 in every 3,500 newborn babies has an underactive thyroid gland, because of failure of the gland to develop normally. In the past, the problem was not recognized until the baby was several weeks old, by which time he or she would have been likely to develop permanent mental and physical handicap—a condition known as cretinism.

Today, however, all babies born in the USA are screened by a blood test (heel-stick test) for hypothyroidism within the first 24 hours after they are born. Any affected babies receive prompt treatment, which ensures that they develop normally. Treatment is with thyroxine and is usually lifelong.

In a few babies, however, the hypothyroidism is temporary, the result of being born to a mother with an underactive thyroid gland; in these women there are blocking antibodies that cross the placenta and that have the opposite effect of the stimulating

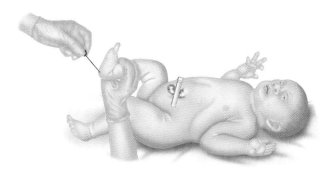

Heel-prick blood test on new baby.

antibodies of Graves' disease and neonatal thyrotoxicosis (see page 75).

Thyroid disease after pregnancy
Graves' disease

Although Graves' disease tends to get better on its own during pregnancy, it often returns—sometimes severely—within a few months of delivery. Treatment of Graves' disease is discussed earlier in this book (see page 26). Unless she is still breast-feeding, the mother can be treated with any of the usual treatments for Graves' disease.

Postpartum thyroiditis

Postpartum (after childbirth) thyroiditis is a form of hyperthyroidism that may develop in the first year after childbirth. It affects up to 5 percent of women, though most are not aware of the symptoms, and may not be treated for it. Most of these women have a tendency towards autoimmune thyroid disease, such as Hashimoto's thyroiditis, though this may not have been recognized previously.

A link has been speculated between postpartum thyroiditis and postpartum depression, but it seems that such a link, if it exists, is actually quite weak.

Usually, the hyperthyroidism is mild and lasts only a few weeks; if treatment proves necessary, a beta-blocker is usually enough. This hyperthyroid phase is usually followed by a transient episode of mild hypothyroidism. Once again, treatment is not usually required, though in a few cases, the symptoms are bad enough that a decision is made to use thyroxine for a few weeks. In almost all cases, the thyroid makes a full recovery, typically after less than 3 to 4 months. A similar pattern may occur in future pregnancies and many patients ultimately develop a permanently underactive thyroid.

Two tests are available to distinguish between postpartum thyroiditis, not requiring treatment, and Graves' disease, which requires treatment.

One is the level of thyroid-stimulating antibody (TRAb) in the blood, as this is usually present in Graves' disease, but absent in postpartum thyroiditis.

The other test is the ability of the thyroid gland to concentrate radioactive iodine or technetium, as this is lacking in postpartum thyroiditis, but present in Graves' disease. Of course, we typically avoid using radioactive tests in women who are breast-feeding.

Case history

Sarah Barkley was 25 when she delivered her first child, a baby girl. A few weeks after the baby was born, Sarah become more emotional than usual, weepy and irritable, snapping at her husband and some of her closest friends for no good reason. She was also sleeping badly and had become shaky and anxious. She put all this down to the hormonal changes following her pregnancy and on "post-partum blues." She assumed that, before long, everything would be back to normal.

However, when she began to complain of palpitations, her husband persuaded her to make an appointment with her family doctor. The doctor thought that Sarah might have an overactive thyroid gland and his suspicions were confirmed by a blood test. On hearing the news, Sarah was concerned because her mother had suffered from Graves' disease when she was in her thirties and her eyes were still very prominent 20 years later, even though the hyperthyroidism had been cured.

To relieve some of her symptoms, Sarah's doctor prescribed propranolol (Inderal™) 40 milligrams twice daily and referred her to an endocrinologist. By the time she saw the endocrinologist, she was already feeling much better and repeat lab work showed that her thyroid gland had become very slightly underactive. The diagnosis was postpartum thyroiditis, and Sarah was reassured that she would not get Graves' Eye Disease like her mother.

The propranolol was stopped and further lab work two months later was entirely normal. Sarah now knows that she may get the symptoms of postpartum thyroiditis after future pregnancies and that she could develop a permanently underactive thyroid gland at some stage in the future. For these reasons, she continues to see her family doctor every year to have her thyroid checked.

KEY POINTS

- If you are being treated for a thyroid problem, tell your doctor if you are planning a pregnancy, or if you become, or think you could be pregnant. You may need a change in your treatment

- If you have a thyroid problem, your thyroid hormone levels should be monitored more closely during pregnancy

- With the right treatment, women with a thyroid problem should have a normal pregnancy. Treatment of a thyroid problem during pregnancy does not put the baby at any increased risk

- Some women will develop thyroid disease after having a baby, but this is usually easy to treat

- Babies born to a mother who has a thyroid problem may have hypothyroidism or hyperthyroidism. This will be detected through routine testing, and the baby can be treated if necessary

Enlarged thyroid (goiter)

Development of a goiter

An enlarged thyroid gland is known as a goiter. Throughout the world, the most common cause of goiter is a deficiency of iodine (page 1), but this is no longer seen in the USA, because iodine is added to many foods and the average North American diet is now quite high in iodine.

Autoimmune disease of the thyroid, including Hashimoto's disease (page 51) and Graves' disease (page 10), often causes a goiter, which may be large enough to be visible in the front of the neck. The cause of many goiters remains unknown, but are thought to be the result of an inherited tendency, often running in families. These are usually called "simple goiter" or "colloid goiter," and the thyroid almost always continues to work normally, even though the gland is larger than usual—the so-called "euthyroid goiter," meaning "a goiter that is making normal amounts of thyroid hormone."

At first, in teenagers and young adults, this goiter is evenly or diffusely enlarged. Over a period of 15 to 25 years, whatever caused the thyroid to grow abnormally in the first place remains and often continues to grow slowly, but becomes lumpy and irregular (nodular), so that by middle age, the goiter will have become a "multinodular goiter."

Simple diffuse goiter

A simple diffuse goiter is most often seen in young women between the ages of 15 and 25. You may notice a symmetrical, smooth swelling in the front of the neck, which moves up and down when you swallow. It is not tender or painful, and usually does not usually cause difficulty in swallowing, though some people experience a tight sensation in the neck.

The goiter may fluctuate in size and be more noticeable during a period or during pregnancy. It isn't normally a problem appearance-wise. In fact, some of the great seventeenth and eighteenth century artists often added a goiter to portraits of women, to make them appear even more beautiful!

Confirming the diagnosis

The first step is making sure that the thyroid is working properly, by checking the TSH and perhaps other thyroid blood tests. To exclude one of the autoimmune thyroid diseases, your physician may check the antibody levels in the blood.

Feeling the shape of the thyroid gland in the neck will confirm that the goiter is diffuse and smooth, with no worrisome nodules. Nowadays, many patients are sent for an ultrasound scan to confirm this, though some physicians still prefer to use a technetium or iodine scan instead of an ultrasound.

Treatment

No treatment is necessary. In the past iodine drops or thyroxine tablets were given, but neither of these approaches works, except when iodine deficiency is the cause of the goiter. In some cases, especially in younger women, the goiter becomes less noticeable or even disappears over a period of a few years.

Simple multinodular goiter

Most patients with a simple multinodular goiter have no symptoms, but discover a lump in the neck by chance, while looking in the mirror. Most people with multinodular goiter are in their forties or older, but the goiter will certainly have been present for many years.

Perhaps the goiter has now reached the critical size of visibility or it may be that your neck has become thinner. Often the goiter is more obvious on one side of the neck than the other, so it may look like a thyroid nodule.

A multinodular goiter can vary in size from being barely visible, to being so large that it becomes embarrassing. A few people hide the goiter by wearing a scarf or high-necked sweater.

Occasionally, a person will first notice the goiter because of the sudden development of pain and swelling in the neck, which is the result of internal bleeding into one of the nodules within the gland. This causes a pain which can sometimes be quite severe, followed by aching discomfort in the neck, like a bruise, lasting several days.

If the goiter becomes very large, there may be difficulty in swallowing dry, solid food. If the trachea (windpipe) is compressed to any extent, the patient can experience breathing difficulty or there may be a change in the voice.

Confirming the diagnosis

A blood sample will confirm that the thyroid is working normally. Because the goiter is nodular, further evaluation is likely be suggested to rule out any worrisome findings. If you are having discomfort or difficulty swallowing, breathing, or speaking, or if the goiter is very large, the endocrinologist may suggest X-rays, a CT scan, breathing tests, or swallowing studies, to determine how much of a problem the goiter is causing. Most of the time, only a few of the following tests are needed.

Breathing tests (pulmonary function tests)

Blowing into a machine can reveal whether the airway is being compressed by the goiter. These tests can also distinguish between the effect of a goiter and some other problem within the lungs causing breathlessness.

CT scan

The CT scan (or CAT scan) is a specialized form of X-ray testing that allows the physician to obtain clear pictures of internal structures in the body. This test is particularly useful for looking at large goiters that lie so low in the neck that they are partly down into the chest. CT scans can be performed either with or without an injection of contrast material. Because the contrast contains large amounts of iodine, most of the time your endocrinologist will ask for the scan to be performed without the contrast, to avoid interfering with other tests of the thyroid.

Swallow study

Swallowing a liquid that shows up on X-rays allows the physician to see whether the goiter is pushing on the

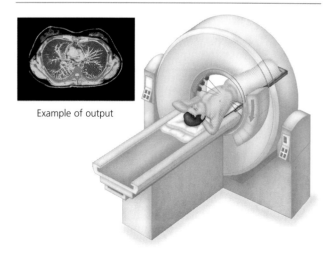

Example of output

Computed tomography (CT) sends X-rays through the body at different angles. The X-rays are picked up by receivers and the information analyzed by a computer to create an anatomical picture.

esophagus (gullet), which might cause swallowing difficulties (dysphagia).

Ultrasound scan
A cold gel is placed on the skin of the front of the neck, and a small hand-held probe is passed over the skin to create an image of the goiter on a computer monitor. As well as showing the size and shape of the goiter, this scan will highlight any cysts or nodules within the gland. It is completely painless.

Isotope scan
This technique provides a picture of the gland that shows whether any of the nodules in the goiter are producing thyroid hormone. If that turns out to be the case, you are at higher risk of developing an overactive

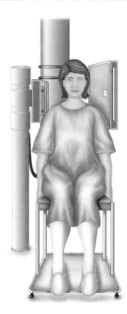

X-ray investigation.

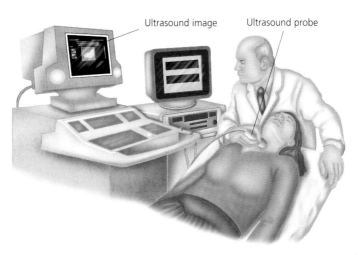

Ultrasound scan.

thyroid in the future. The scan is obtained by injecting a tiny amount of radioactive technetium into a vein, or taking a small dose of radioactive iodine (I-123) by mouth.

An hour or two later, a picture can be taken of the pattern of radioactivity within the thyroid gland. "Hot nodules" are areas of the gland that have taken up the radioactive tracer, and that are likely to be producing thyroid hormone. "Cold nodules" are areas of the gland that are inactive, and have not taken up the tracer. Most cancers form "cold nodules," while "hot nodules" are almost never cancerous.

Fine needle aspiration

Any nodules that look suspiciously cancerous will be biopsied, using a technique called fine needle aspiration biopsy (FNAB). For large nodules that the endocrinologist can feel, this technique can be performed in the doctor's office. For smaller nodules, the FNAB is usually performed using the guidance of an ultrasound machine, which allows the needle to be placed into the nodule under direct vision. The ultrasound-guided FNAB used to be performed only in a hospital radiology department, but nowadays many endocrinologists have an ultrasound machine in their own office, and will perform the biopsy at the same time that you are being evaluated for the goiter.

The biopsy is performed by placing a fine needle— usually smaller than that used to draw a blood sample from your arm—through the skin of the neck, and into the thyroid nodule. Most of the time, an anesthetic is not needed, though some lidocaine can be injected into the skin, if necessary, to numb the area. By applying suction to the needle when it is inside the nodule, some of the

Fine needle aspiration

The doctor extracts cells from the thyroid gland using a syringe with a fine needle.

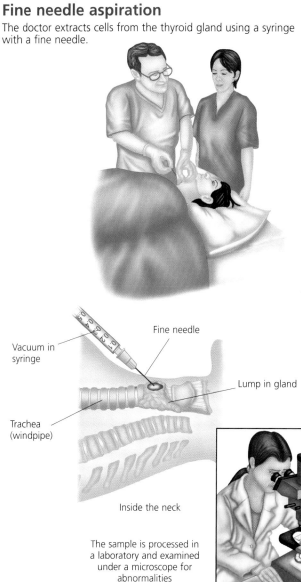

Fine needle

Vacuum in syringe

Lump in gland

Trachea (windpipe)

Inside the neck

The sample is processed in a laboratory and examined under a microscope for abnormalities

cells can be withdrawn, spread onto a glass slide, and analyzed by a pathologist to determine the nature of the nodule. Typically, an endocrinologist will insert the needle into the nodule between three and six times, to ensure enough cells are available for the Pathologist to analyze.

Most patients find the FNAB to be uncomfortable, but not particularly painful. Complications are usually limited to a little bruising on the front of the neck. Very rarely, infection or significant bleeding has been reported as a complication of FNAB, but these problems are exceptionally rare, and the procedure is extremely safe.

Most of the time, the FNAB provides an accurate diagnosis within a few hours, or a day or two. There is a further discussion of FNAB results later in this book, on page 98 (Thyroid nodules).

Treatment

If your goiter is small, you probably won't need any treatment. Regular checks of your TSH every one to two years are important, because the gland may become overactive and cause hyperthyroidism at some stage in later life, often 20 years or more later.

Thyroxine treatment is still used occasionally to try to shrink the goiter, but this is no longer recommended as it rarely works, and can cause side effects if it results in hyperthyroidism.

Surgery

If the goiter enlarges to the point that it becomes unsightly, or if it starts to compress the trachea or the esophagus, or if it begins to affect the voice, the most effective treatment is surgery to remove most of the thyroid gland.

The surgical technique, the risk of complications, and the outcome of surgery are identical to the surgery that is used for Graves' disease or TMNG, discussed on page 14. After this type of surgery, you will develop hypothyroidism, which will require lifelong treatment with thyroid hormone.

Radioactive iodine

Radioactive iodine is sometimes used instead of surgery, but it is less likely to be helpful unless the gland has also become overactive (see TMNG, page 14). A large dose of radioactive iodine is often necessary, sometimes requiring admission to hospital for 24–48 hours to allow the radioactivity to fall to safe levels. Some shrinkage of the goiter is likely, but it may take several months to become fully effective.

In an effort to improve this technique, some endocrinologists are experimenting with using injections of recombinant human TSH (rhTSH; Thyrogen™) to increase the efficiency of the gland's uptake of iodine. This approach has some promise, but is currently experimental and has not been approved by the FDA at this time. A more detailed discussion of rhTSH starts on page 117.

Case history

Mary Harrison lived alone and was 84 years old when she developed gallstones and was admitted to the local hospital for surgery. She had always worn a silk scarf around her neck, day and night, summer and winter. Friends and neighbors thought it was part of her slightly eccentric personality, but when the scarf was removed in hospital, she was forced to reveal a large goiter and a scar from a previous thyroid operation.

She explained to the resident that the operation had been for a goiter when she was in her twenties, but by her mid-forties the goiter had appeared again. She was told then that further surgery was impossible, because a second operation might damage the nerve supply to the voice-box (larynx) and damage her voice. Gradually, the goiter had grown larger and she took to wearing the scarves to avoid embarrassment.

Blood tests in hospital showed her to have a slightly overactive thyroid gland, so she was treated with radioactive iodine. Two months later, her lab tests showed her thyroid had returned to normal, and over the next several months the size of the goiter decreased considerably.

Although she was reassured that more surgery was possible—and safe—if performed by an experienced surgeon, she preferred to avoid an operation for another few years, in case her goiter grew again in the future. She reassured her doctors that she would get back to them "in another twenty years or so"!

Thyroid nodules

Lumps or nodules in the thyroid are very common, affecting as many as one in every five people in the USA. Using an ultrasound scan to check the thyroid gland shows that small thyroid nodules are even more common than this, affecting as many as half of all women over the age of 50 years. Of course, almost all of these nodules are benign and non-cancerous.

The main problem with small thyroid nodules is trying to decide which ones to worry about and which ones to ignore—looking for thyroid cancer is like looking for a needle in a haystack! For larger nodules—again they are almost always benign—the difficulty is

The possible change of a goiter over a lifetime

The smooth simple goiter of young adulthood changes to the multinodular goiter of middle age and the toxic multinodular goiter of old age. The cause of the goiter is not known but, if whatever makes the thyroid gland grow in the first place continues to be present, the thyroid can develop lumps or nodules. These nodules make their own thyroid hormones and, as they increase in number and size over many years, hyperthyroidism develops. The windpipe (trachea), shown by the dotted lines, may be displaced and narrowed as the goiter enlarges.

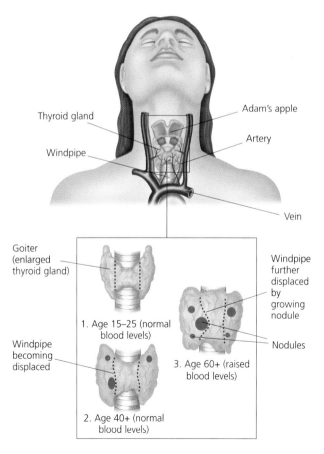

Thyroid gland

Windpipe

Adam's apple

Artery

Vein

Goiter (enlarged thyroid gland)

Windpipe becoming displaced

1. Age 15–25 (normal blood levels)

2. Age 40+ (normal blood levels)

Windpipe further displaced by growing nodule

Nodules

3. Age 60+ (raised blood levels)

deciding whether the lump is big enough to be worth removing surgically: swapping a lump for a scar.

A single thyroid nodule

Nodules can sometimes be felt when they are as small as a pea, but sometimes they can be missed until they are the size of a golf ball or even larger. Most people with a thyroid nodule discover it by accident while looking in a mirror. Others have a nodule discovered during a routine physical, when the physician examines the neck.

To check out your own thyroid gland, stand in front of a mirror with your head tilted slightly backward and the neck stretched. Take a small sip of water and watch your neck as you swallow. The thyroid gland lies an inch or two below the Adam's apple and a little off to each side. If you have a small goiter, or a thyroid nodule, you may be able to see it move up and then down again as you swallow. If you do this and find a lump, make sure you have it checked by your physician!

Currently, more and more thyroid nodules are being found during tests being performed for some completely unrelated problem. These tests can include chest X-rays (though usually only very large masses are found this way), CT scans, MRI scans, PET scans, and ultrasound scans.

The finding of a lump always leads to fear of the possibility of cancer. While it is true that most thyroid cancer causes a lump in the thyroid gland, it's important to remember that almost always a lump in the thyroid turns out NOT to be a cancer. Only about one in every 2,000 thyroid nodules eventually proves to be a thyroid cancer.

Confirming the diagnosis

If you have a thyroid nodule, the blood work will usually show normal levels of TSH, T_4, and T_3, and you will be classified medically as "euthyroid' (meaning "normal thyroid function"). The exception is a "toxic adenoma," a nodule that is actively making thyroid hormone, in which the thyroid tests show a low TSH, diagnosing an overactive thyroid gland. In this case, almost all of the thyroid hormone is coming from the nodule, while the rest of the thyroid will be shut down.

If the TSH is low you will be recommended to have a radioactive isotope scan and uptake measurement (usually with technetium and/or radioactive iodine; see page 93), to confirm that the hyperthyroidism is being caused by the nodule. In these cases, the nodule is always benign and treatment can be undertaken safely with either surgery or radioactive iodine, as described for TMNG above (page 93).

For patients with a nodule that is not overactive, the crucial question is whether the nodule could be cancerous. The endocrinologist will examine your neck carefully, because almost half of all patients thought to have a single nodule are, in fact, found to have multiple nodules, as part of a multinodular goiter (page 14). These nodules are almost always completely benign and require no further testing.

For patients with a true solitary nodule, or a nodular gland in which the main nodule is out of keeping with the rest of the thyroid gland, further testing will be suggested. In the past, a radioisotope scan was the preferred first test, to distinguish a "cold" nodule (inactive, not taking up the radioactive iodine or technetium) from a "hot" nodule (active, taking up the tracer). Only the cold nodules would then be evaluated, because cancer always causes a cold nodule. Unfortunately, this test is not a particularly useful one, because most of those cold nodules were, in fact, still benign. In addition, this type of scan is quite insensitive, with many smaller nodules not showing up at all on the scan.

Nowadays, an ultrasound scan is the preferred way to look at thyroid nodules. In many cases, the ultrasound machine will be available in the endocrinologist's office, so that having the scan does not require a separate appointment with the radiologist.

If a solitary nodule is confirmed on ultrasound, or if the nodule is particularly large, you will be advised to be subjected to a fine needle aspiration biopsy (FNAB) of the lump. This technique is described on page 107. FNAB is one of the most useful and accurate tests in the management of thyroid nodules.

In the past, most patients with a thyroid nodule had to have surgery simply to make sure the lump was benign, which most were, leading to a lot of unnecessary surgery. Many of these operations can now be avoided simply by performing a FNAB in the office. Within a few hours or a day or two, after the pathologist has finished studying the slides, the results become available. Those results will be one of the following.

Benign

Sometimes the report reads "consistent with a benign thyroid nodule," which means the same thing. The nodule is not cancer, it is not pre-cancerous, and will not turn into cancer. This is a very reassuring finding. If the FNAB is done properly and the results are interpreted by an expert pathologist, this result is as accurate as any test in medicine can ever be. Missing a cancer is almost unheard of, unless the nodule was tiny and the needle missed the cancerous area.

Malignant

The cells removed show strong evidence that this nodule is a cancer of the thyroid. Once again, this result is very reliable, and although the news is not good, at least you will now know that this nodule needs to be treated seriously. You will need surgery and may require other treatment too, as described in the chapter on Thyroid cancer (pages 103–127)

Suspicious

Sometimes the report reads "suspicious for follicular neoplasm." The cells removed are suspicious and may represent a cancer or a pre-cancerous nodule. With this type of result, surgery is necessary, though only about one in three to one in five of these nodules actually turns out to contain cancer. Often the surgeon will remove only half of the gland, to obtain a more accurate report from the pathologist, before deciding whether a more extensive surgery is going to be needed.

Non-diagnostic

If the biopsy specimen did not capture enough cells, it may be impossible for the pathologist to be certain whether the nodule is benign or malignant. In this case, your endocrinologist may recommend repeating the biopsy, perhaps using a larger biopsy needle. In some cases, the problem is just that there was fluid within the nodule (a cyst), in which case, your endocrinologist may suggest simply watching the area with the ultrasound and repeating the biopsy only if the problem comes back. Sometimes, if your endocrinologist is concerned that this might actually be a cancer, he or she will recommend surgery to remove the nodule, just as if the biopsy report had been "suspicious"

Benign (non-cancerous) nodules can continue to enlarge over the years and sometimes become big enough for surgery to be needed to remove them, either for appearance's sake, or because the nodule is causing pressure symptoms in the neck. Fortunately, this is unusual.

A few people continue to worry that a lump could be cancerous, even though the FNAB was reassuring. For these individuals, it may be best simply to have the nodule removed. While this may not be medically strictly necessary, it is still reasonable for some people, since the surgery is generally very safe.

Except when dealing with a nodule that is known to be cancerous, the normal surgery to remove a thyroid nodule is removal of the lobe (half of the thyroid) that contains the nodule. The reason for this is that efforts to shell out the nodule from the gland make the pathologist's job much harder, leading to an inaccurate final pathology report. In addition, removal of a thyroid lobe (lobectomy) is generally a safer operation than removal of a lump from within the gland, with less chance of bleeding.

After a thyroid lobectomy, the patient still has half of the thyroid gland left in place. In most cases (more than 80 percent), the remaining thyroid is able to increase its production of thyroid hormone and keep up with the body's demands. Although a few patients suffer mild hypothyroidism after the surgery, most will recover within just a few weeks and then have normal thyroid function for the remainder of their lives.

KEY POINTS

- Most goiters in the USA are either "simple goiter" or multinodular goiters. The cause of both remains a mystery

- Young people with a simple diffuse goiter do not need any treatment

- The finding of a goiter needs further investigation, involving blood tests, a thorough examination of the thyroid gland, and possibly an ultrasound scan. Larger goiters may need more sophisticated testing performed by an endocrinologist

- A small multinodular goiter may not require any treatment, but regular tests are needed in case hyperthyroidism develops subsequently

- If the goiter becomes overactive, causing hyperthyroidism, either surgery or radioactive iodine can be used

- Large goiters may need to be removed surgically

- Thyroxine treatment rarely helps to shrink a goiter, and side effects can be a problem

- Thyroid nodules are very common, and most turn out not to be cancerous or pre-cancerous

- Evaluation of a solitary thyroid nodule involves a fine needle aspiration biopsy (FNAB), which is sometimes performed with an ultrasound to guide the needle into the right place

- Surgery to remove a thyroid nodule should be considered if the nodule is cancerous, suspicious, or if it is simply big enough to be a nuisance. Thyroid surgery is also used if a nodule is unsightly, or if either the patient or the endocrinologist is worried about the possibility of cancer

Thyroid cancer

What is cancer?

All human tissues are made up of billions of cells, visible only through a microscope. These cells function in harmony to perform the normal functions of the human body. Most cells live for a relatively short time, while new cells grow to replace those lost through old-age and wear and tear.

A piece of human tissue the size of a dime may contain a thousand million cells. These are the minute building blocks from which our bodies are made, visible only down the microscope. It is quite amazing that the billions of cells in a human body normally function in perfect harmony, every cell knowing its place and doing the job that it was designed to do. Most cells have a finite lifespan: millions of new ones are produced every day to replace those lost through old age or wear and tear.

New cells are produced when existing cells divide into two. Except in children, who are growing, there is normally a perfect balance between the numbers of the cells that are dying and those that are being formed. Normally exactly the right number of new cells are produced to replace those that are being lost. The

How a tumor forms

A cancerous tumor begins as a single cell. If it is not destroyed by the body's immune system, it will double into two cells, which in turn divide into four and so on.

Cancerous cell

First doubling

Second doubling

control mechanisms involved are exceedingly complex, complicated and not yet fully understood. What we do know is that, when something goes wrong with those controls, too many cells can be created, forming a tumor.

However, it is important to realize that only a small minority of tumors are cancerous. Most tumors are localized accumulations of normal or fairly normal cells and are benign. A wart is a common example.

The development of a cancer (malignant tumor) involves a change in the quality of the cells as well as an increase in quantity: they change in both appearance and behavior. They become more aggressive, destructive, and independent of normal cells. They acquire the ability to infiltrate and invade the surrounding tissues.

In some instances the cells may also invade lymphatic and blood vessels and use these routes to spread away from the "primary" growth to other places. In time these cells may cause the development of secondary growths, known as "metastases," in the lymph glands and other organs such as lungs, liver and bones.

How cancer spreads

Cancerous tumors can spread to distant sites in the body by a process called metastasis. In metastasis the cancerous cell separates from a malignant tumor and travels to a new location in the blood or lymph.

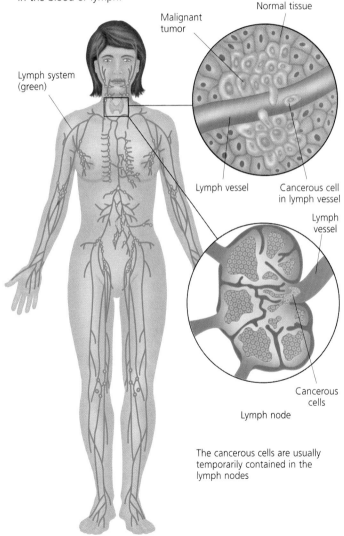

Malignant tumor

Normal tissue

Lymph system (green)

Lymph vessel

Cancerous cell in lymph vessel

Lymph vessel

Cancerous cells

Lymph node

The cancerous cells are usually temporarily contained in the lymph nodes

Thyroid cancer

Cancer of the thyroid is rare; there are only about 30,000 cases each year in the USA, out of a population of almost 300 million people (roughly one case in every 10,000 people). Because thyroid cancer causes a lump in the neck, which is often visible or easy to feel, most thyroid cancers are discovered at an early stage, when they can be treated and often cured. In fact, of all cancers, thyroid cancer is one of the most likely to be curable. For young people in particular, thyroid cancer generally has an excellent prognosis, as long as it is properly treated.

There are four major types of thyroid cancer:

- Papillary thyroid cancer, the most common type, accounting for more than eight out of 10 thyroid cancers in the USA.
- Follicular thyroid cancer, most often seen in people in their thirties and forties.
- Medullary thyroid cancer, a rare type of thyroid cancer that sometimes runs in families.
- Anaplastic thyroid cancer, an aggressive and dangerous type, which fortunately is extremely rare.

The names of these cancer types describe the appearance of the tumor under the microscope. In papillary cancer, the tumor contains "papillae" or fronds, whereas in follicular cancer, although the appearance is distinctly abnormal, the structures still resemble the normal follicles of the thyroid gland.

Both of these common types of thyroid cancer can occur at any age, but patients with papillary cancer tend to be a little younger than people with follicular cancer. Women are affected with thyroid cancer about 3–4 times more often than men, though it is not known why. Most thyroid cancers do not appear to run in families, though occasionally a family could have more than one person affected with any of these cancer types. Medullary cancer is found to be familial in about 20% of cases, so genetic testing and family screening are recommended for anyone related to a patient suffering from this form of thyroid cancer. Anaplastic cancer most often develops in older people (usually over 60 years old), especially those who have had a goiter or other thyroid problem for many years. It is a very dangerous and often lethal form of cancer, for which treatment is only rarely successful.

Confirming the diagnosis

Most patients are diagnosed with thyroid cancer after finding a lump in the neck, or because of rapid growth of a goiter, which they may have known about for years. The diagnosis of thyroid cancer is typically made by fine needle aspiration biopsy (FNAB), or at the time of thyroid surgery for removal of a nodule or a goiter.

Less frequently, the first finding of a thyroid cancer is made because of enlarged lymph nodes in the neck, nodes that turn out to contain thyroid cancer that has spread from the primary tumor in the thyroid gland. Rather surprisingly, unlike many other cancer types, thyroid cancer that has spread to the lymph nodes is still usually very treatable, and the prognosis remains excellent in most cases.

Treatment
Surgery
Thyroid cancer is almost always best treated by removing the cancer along with as much of the thyroid gland as possible (what is known as a near-total or

Microscopic view of the thyroid gland

The follicles seen here in cross-section resemble small golf balls. The dimples in the surface correspond to the follicle cells that make thyroid hormones and release them into the capillaries, which lie close by. The colloid is like the semi-liquid filling of old-fashioned golf balls, a gel-like substance, which contains reserves of thyroid hormone. There are many thousands of follicles in a thyroid gland. The superimposed needle tip shows the process of fine needle aspiration, during which a small sample of cells is obtained for microscopic analysis.

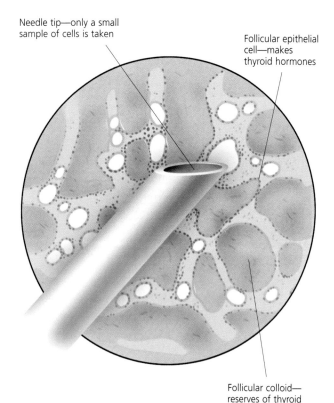

Needle tip—only a small sample of cells is taken

Follicular epithelial cell—makes thyroid hormones

Follicular colloid— reserves of thyroid hormone are stored here

total thyroidectomy). For very small cancers that have not spread beyond one side of the thyroid, some surgeons prefer to remove only the half of the thyroid (lobectomy) that contains the cancer, to reduce the risk of complications.

In a near-total thyroidectomy, a tiny amount of thyroid tissue is left behind to protect the other structures in the neck, particularly the recurrent laryngeal nerves that control the larynx (voice box), and the parathyroid glands that regulate calcium in the blood. The outcome of near-total and total thyroidectomy is the same, and most surgeons will achieve 98–100% removal of the gland with either of these operations.

Any lymph nodes in the neck containing thyroid cancer will also be removed at the time of the surgery. In fact, it is very common for some lymph nodes to be found to contain cancer at the time of the surgery, particularly in papillary thyroid cancer, but it is important to realize that this is not a particularly dangerous or worrisome sign in this type of cancer.

In order to identify cancerous lymph nodes, it is usual to obtain an ultrasound scan of the neck before performing the surgery. This allows the surgeon to see a map of where the cancerous nodes might be, and to adjust the surgery if necessary.

If the lymph nodes lie around and close to the thyroid, then the surgical incision is very similar to that used in surgery for Graves' disease, discussed earlier (page 10), i.e., a low neck incision, usually in a skin crease, measuring 2 or 3 inches in length. If the cancer has already spread into lymph nodes further out in the neck, a longer incision might be needed, following along the line of the carotid artery in the neck.

Typically, surgery for thyroid cancer takes between

2 and 4 hours, and most patients leave the hospital after only one overnight stay. Complications can arise, of course, but they are rare, particularly if the surgeon is experienced.

Damage to the parathyroid glands causes a fall in the blood calcium levels, which may need treatment with a strong version of Vitamin D (Rocaltrol™ or Calcitriol™).

Damage to the recurrent laryngeal nerve is also possible, but rare unless the cancer has already invaded, injured, or destroyed the nerve. Damage to this nerve causes hoarseness and a change in the voice. It can also create a problem with breathing, but only if both nerves are damaged, which fortunately is a very rare event. Bruising of the nerve happens quite commonly, however, leading to temporary hoarseness, but recovery usually only takes a matter of weeks.

Similarly, bruising and injury to the parathyroid glands can cause a drop in the calcium level, which requires short-term treatment with vitamin D and calcium, again usually for just a few weeks.

Other complications include bleeding, bruising, and infection. Other nerve injury in the neck is very rare, and would only be anticipated if the cancer is very extensive, leading to a much bigger operation.

Radioactive iodine

Radioactive iodine can be a useful way to kill thyroid tissue, including a cancerous thyroid. Unfortunately, it cannot be used as an alternative to surgery, because too much of the tumor would need to be destroyed and too much of the radioactivity would be absorbed by the normal thyroid gland, making it ineffective in killing the cancer. Radioactive iodine can be useful, however, in treating thyroid cancer that, for one reason or another, cannot be removed by surgery alone.

If the cancer has already spread to other organs by the time it is diagnosed (metastatic disease), radioactive iodine can sometimes be used to seek out and destroy the thyroid cancer. This treatment is given only after the thyroid gland itself, as well as the primary thyroid cancer, has been removed.

Radioactive iodine is most effective in treating young patients with papillary thyroid cancer, whose disease has spread into the lungs. This is a rare event, but having radioactive iodine available as a treatment for these patients is very useful. Although the dose of radioactivity used is quite high, the risk of the radiation is actually very low, and it may prove to be life-saving, because no other effective way of killing metastatic thyroid cancer is known.

Radioactive iodine is also used frequently to try to destroy deposits of thyroid cancer contained in the lymph nodes of the neck. Although radioactive iodine is often taken up into those lymph nodes, it may not be quite so effective in destroying cancer deposits, and surgery to remove the lymph nodes involved may be necessary if the radioactive iodine does not work. For this reason, removal of cancerous lymph nodes should always be undertaken at the time of the original thyroid surgery.

Increasingly in the USA, and around the world, endocrinologists are using radioactive iodine to "ablate" (remove) remaining normal thyroid tissue after the surgery, even for patients in whom the thyroid cancer has been successfully cut out using surgery. Endocrinologists who promote this approach—known as "remnant ablation"—argue that radioactive iodine is safe (though they will probably place the patient in isolation in a lead-lined room for 24–48 hours after administering the treatment). The reason for this procedure is that some cancerous thyroid cancer cells may still be "hiding out" in the neck, or elsewhere, even after surgery, and this ensures that they are destroyed.

Although the idea that we might "cure" thyroid cancer better by following surgery with radioactive iodine treatment routinely is an attractive one, there is actually very little evidence to support this approach, at least in young people with papillary thyroid cancer. In such cases, the outlook is so good with surgery alone (a normal life expectancy) that it is unlikely that the outcome could be any better with additional treatment. Careful studies have shown that routine radioactive iodine treatment does not improve the chances of avoiding a recurrence of the disease in the future. Monitoring will be necessary in any case, as discussed later in this chapter.

Finally, there is now very convincing evidence that radioactive iodine in the high doses used for thyroid cancer treatment and even for remnant ablation actually carries a small but significant risk of causing cancers of other types. These cancers include endometrial and ovarian cancer in women, and colon, salivary gland, and bone cancers in both men and women. As usual in medicine, side effects can result from any procedure, and radioactive iodine is no exception. It is very important that you and your endocrinologist weigh the risks and the benefits of radioactive iodine before going ahead with this treatment.

The American Thyroid Association, one of the world's leading professional organizations for specialists in diseases of the thyroid, recently convened a committee of experts to advise endocrinologists on the use of radioactive iodine (as well as other treatments) in the management of thyroid cancer.

The committee recommended that patients with Stage 1 papillary and follicular thyroid cancer should be treated with radioactive iodine "only in selected cases," particularly if there was something unusual about their cancer. To put this in perspective, it is worth knowing that more than 60% of patients—almost two out of every three—with thyroid cancer are diagnosed in Stage I of the disease! According to the committee, only a minority of thyroid cancer patients need treatment with radioactive iodine. You can find more detailed information on these treatment guidelines at the American Thyroid Association website: www.thyroid.org.

If you are given radioactive iodine treatment, it will normally be administered 6–8 weeks after the thyroid surgery. To give the cancer the best chance to take up the radioactive iodine, it is important for you to be hypothyroid at the time. This can be achieved by stopping your thyroid hormone at least four weeks before the treatment is given.

During this time, you may develop at least some of the symptoms of hypothyroidism (see pages 51–71). To decrease the length of time you suffer from these symptoms, some endocrinologists suggest using T_3 treatment (Cytomel™) for the first four weeks after stopping thyroxine, followed by two weeks off all thyroid hormones, before undergoing radioactive iodine treatment. Because T_3 is a short-acting hormone, two weeks is usually enough to allow the body to become hypothyroid and to increase the TSH level to the range that is best for the radioactive iodine treatment. Most endocrinologists like to see the TSH level rise to at least 30 mU/L before administering radioactive iodine treatment.

During this time, you will likely be recommended to follow a diet low in iodine. This causes short-term iodine deficiency, which is not harmful, but which gives the cancer the best chance to take up and be killed by the radioactive iodine you then receive. Although a low-iodine diet can be unpleasant to follow closely, remember that it is only necessary for a few weeks before treatment.

Radioactive iodine is administered as a liquid or a capsule, most often in hospital. For high doses (the recommended limits vary from state to state), you will have to stay in hospital for 24–48 hours, in isolation, until the radiation levels in the body fall to those that are regarded as safe for people around you.

If you receive the treatment as an outpatient, you will be given very clear instructions about what you can and cannot do for several days after the treatment. In general, the aim of these rules is to keep others around you safe and to avoid contaminating them with unnecessary radiation.

You will be advised to avoid public places, such as movie theaters and restaurants, and close and intimate contact with your partner or with young children. You will have to stay away from work if your work involves food preparation or dealing with children or the general public. These restrictions remain in place for a number of days, depending on the dose of radioactive iodine you have received.

After you have been treated with radioactive iodine, your thyroxine can be re-started in full dosage within a few days. You will start to notice the symptoms of hypothyroidism reduce and disappear within 10 to 14 days.

Thyroxine suppressive therapy

The growth rate of papillary and follicular cancers can be accelerated by high levels of TSH. Keeping the TSH level low is therefore a sensible part of the treatment for thyroid cancer. To achieve this, you will typically be prescribed a dose of thyroid hormone that is a little higher than your body expects. The dose is then adjusted ("titrated") until the level of TSH in your blood falls to a point slightly below the normal range. In other words, your endocrinologist is trying to give you a very mild case of hyperthyroidism.

The dose needed for TSH suppression is generally slightly higher than the dose of thyroxine needed to keep the TSH normal, which is the goal of treatment for hypothyroidism. On average, the required dose is between 150 and 200 mcg, though some people need less and others much more. Because the goal of treatment is to keep the TSH low without causing excessive symptoms of hyperthyroidism, it is particularly important that you take the medication regularly, reliably, and appropriately, along the lines discussed in the chapter on hypothyroidism (pages 51–71).

This slight over-treatment with thyroxine can sometimes cause mild symptoms of hyperthyroidism. Most patients, however, notice nothing more than a slightly faster heart rate, a few minor palpitations, or a little sensitivity to heat. In most cases, these symptoms are very mild, and fade slowly as the body adapts to the higher-than-normal thyroid hormone levels. Symptoms that are troublesome should always be discussed with your endocrinologist, as some people simply cannot tolerate these high doses. So long as the risk from cancer is felt to be low, some people's cases are better managed by keeping the TSH within the normal range, but toward the low end of that range.

Older patients receiving treatment with these higher doses of thyroxine may be at slightly increased risk of developing osteoporosis (especially women) or atrial fibrillation. Careful attention to these possibilities is one of the reasons why follow-up with an endocrinologist is strongly recommended for people with thyroid cancer.

The goal of thyroxine suppressive therapy of this type is to give any remaining thyroid cancer cells a disadvantage, and to give your body an advantage in fighting the cancer. There is evidence that a healthy young adult can contain, control, and even destroy tiny remnants of thyroid cancer in this way. The usual recommendation is to keep the TSH level slightly suppressed for at least the first 3–5 years after surgery. After that, assuming there has been no recurrence of the cancer, the dose of thyroid hormone can usually be reduced a little, allowing the TSH to be returned to the normal range.

Follow-up

Several strategies for following up thyroid cancer are available. The ideal follow-up strategy depends on the type of thyroid cancer you had, the stage of the cancer when it was detected, and whether the treatment was felt to have been successful.

Thyroglobulin

Papillary and follicular cancers, like the normal thyroid gland, make a protein called thyroglobulin, which is released into the bloodstream, and which can be detected by a laboratory test. If thyroglobulin is detected in the bloodstream, then there must be thyroid tissue—either normal or cancerous—somewhere in the body. As a result, after thyroid surgery, measurement of thyroglobulin provides a useful means of detecting a recurrence of thyroid cancer.

It is important to remember that, even after surgery and radioactive iodine treatment, some small amount of normal thyroid tissue often remains. As a result, a low detectable level of thyroglobulin does not always mean that cancer is still present. Many patients have a low level in the blood that stays stable over many years, or gradually reduces and disappears. In these people, the thyroglobulin is almost certainly coming from a tiny remnant of normal thyroid tissue.

More worrisome would be a level of thyroglobulin that keeps rising in test after test. In those cases, finding and treating the source of the thyroglobulin is important.

Recombinant human TSH (rhTSH, Thyrogen™)

Recombinant human TSH is a protein identical to TSH from the pituitary gland, but which has been made in the laboratory through a form of genetic engineering. This artificial hormone can be given by intramuscular injection and is absorbed quickly into the bloodstream where it acts in the same way as your own TSH.

Administering two injections of this drug, on two consecutive days, causes the TSH level to rise to levels similar to those that would occur after stopping thyroxine treatment for several weeks. Using rhTSH in this way, however, avoids the symptoms of hypothyroidism that affect people who stop taking thyroxine for a period of time.

TSH (both the natural form and rhTSH) stimulates thyroglobulin production from normal thyroid tissue and thyroid cancer tissue. As a result, withdrawing thyroid hormone for a few weeks to allow the TSH to rise, or giving shots of recombinant human TSH (rhTSH), can cause a previously undetectable thyroglobulin to become detectable. This finding increases the sensitivity of detection of thyroid tissue, though it does not help to distinguish thyroglobulin produced by a cancer from that produced by a normal thyroid tissue remnant.

Whether this stimulated thyroglobulin measurement is a necessary part of your follow-up for thyroid cancer should be determined depending on the type and stage of thyroid cancer you had, and by your endocrinologist's level of concern that your cancer might not have been cured.

Both thyroid hormone withdrawal and rhTSH injections can also be used to perform whole body radioactive iodine scans, which are also part of the follow-up for some patients with thyroid cancer. At the present time, however, rhTSH is not approved by the FDA to prepare patients for treatment with radioactive iodine, either for thyroid tissue remnant ablation or for treatment of known thyroid cancer, because the radioactive iodine treatment may not be quite as effective when performed this way.

Whole body iodine scan

Across the USA, whole body iodine scans remain one of the main forms of follow-up for patients with

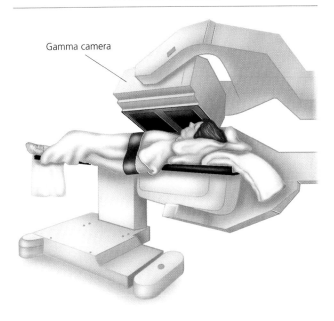

Gamma camera

Whole body scan using radioactive iodine and a gamma camera.

thyroid cancer. These scans rely on the fact that thyroid cancer is often capable of taking up iodine. Giving a dose of radioactive iodine (either I-123 or I-131) by mouth allows this radiation to be taken up by any remaining thyroid tissue and the iodine can then be detected using cameras sensitive to radiation.

A whole body iodine scan is usually performed after a few weeks of a low-iodine diet, to gain the maximum sensitivity for the test. In addition, the TSH level must be high enough to encourage the thyroid tissue (or thyroid cancer) to take up the iodine. This can be achieved either by withdrawing thyroid hormone (in exactly the same way as described for treatment with radioactive iodine on page 93), or by injecting rhTSH intramuscularly on two consecutive days, 24–48 hours before giving the radioactive iodine tracer dose. The tracer is then given by mouth and a scan is performed 24 hours later.

In addition to thyroid tissue, the radioactive iodine is taken up into the saliva glands, the stomach, colon, kidneys, and bladder. Areas of significant uptake elsewhere should indicate the presence of thyroid tissue, including thyroid cancer.

Whole body scans are a useful way to identify thyroid cancer that takes up iodine, particularly if that cancer has spread outside the thyroid into other organs. The scans are not as sensitive as we might wish, sometimes missing small areas of cancer, particularly in lymph nodes in the neck. However, in conjunction with measurement of thyroglobulin, they are a good way to follow patients at high risk for recurrence of thyroid cancer.

Ultrasound Scan

Because most patients who suffer a recurrence of thyroid cancer are found to have that cancer contained in lymph nodes in the neck, one of the most successful ways of monitoring these patients is with an ultrasound scan.

This is probably the most sensitive test for studying the lymph nodes in the neck, and can often find abnormal lymph nodes when no other scan shows any signs of thyroid cancer. In fact, sometimes the scan is so sensitive that it detects tiny deposits of thyroid cancer only a millimeter or two in size.

The problem then is how to deal with those deposits, because in many cases, radioactive iodine does not eliminate these tiny cancer deposits, and surgery on the neck seems like using a hammer to crack a nut!

Even so, the ultrasound scan is quickly becoming the investigation of first choice in monitoring patients with thyroid cancer, particularly as more and more endocrinologists and radiologists are gaining familiarity with this very powerful tool.

Other types of scan (CT, MRI, PET)

Imaging of the neck, chest, and other parts of the body can be an important tool in the follow-up of some patients, particularly those in whom the cancer has already spread, or in whom the risks of it spreading are felt to be high. Once again, the details of follow-up depend very much on the type of thyroid cancer and the stage at which it was diagnosed. CT scans are particularly good for looking inside the chest and abdomen. MRI scans are better for investigating the brain and other solid organs, such as the liver and adrenal glands. PET scanning is also being used more frequently for tracking disease that has spread widely—fortunately a rare event in most types of thyroid cancer.

Prognosis

The prognosis in thyroid cancer depends on the age of the patient (younger is better), the size of the tumor (smaller is better), whether it has spread at the time of diagnosis, and whether the surgeon is able to remove all of the cancer. Somewhat surprisingly, the prognosis, at least for papillary cancer, the most common type, does not seem to alter if the cancer has spread into the lymph nodes of the neck, though it can be harder to completely eradicate the disease.

There are several very accurate ways to determine the prognosis of a patient with thyroid cancer, but the most widely used is to determine the Stage the disease has reached. Most endocrinologists use this and other similar systems to try to get a better handle on a patient's prognosis. Knowing, for example, that a patient has a small low-risk papillary thyroid cancer at a young age will allow the endocrinologist to reassure that person, while avoiding potentially harmful treatments, and to use a follow-up strategy geared toward the needs of that patient. Alternatively, thyroid cancer in an older patient who has a higher-risk, more aggressive type of cancer, may well spread to other organs; it can now be identified, treated more vigorously, and followed up more intensely.

Fortunately, most people with thyroid cancer contract the low risk form of the disease and as a result have a normal life expectancy, with a very low risk of problems arising from the cancer.

Treatment of recurrent thyroid cancer

Thyroid cancer is supposed to be curable, so it is particularly frightening when a patient is told that the disease is back. Fortunately, in most cases, this is not really a recurrence of the disease in the true sense of the word. In most cases, what has been discovered is residual (left over) disease, which was contained within lymph nodes of the neck, but was too small to be seen at the time of the surgery.

In these cases, treatment with radioactive iodine might be effective, though more surgery is sometimes needed to clear the cancer. For very small deposits of cancer within one or two lymph nodes, simple observation may be worthwhile instead, because there is a reasonable chance that these deposits will be stabilized, contained, or even destroyed by the body's immune system.

Alternatively, a small number of centers around the country have developed non-surgical treatment alternatives, including the injection of medical alcohol (ethanol ablation), freezing the cancer tissue (cryo-ablation) or high-frequency microwaves (radiofrequency ablation).

These techniques are highly specialized, available only in a few centers, and may be applicable only to selected patients. They may be worth exploring, however, if other options for treatment seem not to be working, or are felt to be too risky. Your endocrinologist will be able to refer you to one of the large medical centers that perform these techniques, if necessary.

For patients with disease that has spread beyond the neck, radioactive iodine treatment is the only treatment that has proven to be effective. If radioactive iodine fails, it is common to use external beam radiation therapy (X-ray therapy) for threatening areas of disease. This approach can be useful for cancer deposits in the neck—if no other treatment is available—or in the bones. Radiation therapy does have significant side-effects, however, including skin burns, scar formation and damage to surrounding organs, so it is generally reserved for situations where the tumor is threatening vital functions and cannot be treated any other way.

For other sites of tumor spread, chemotherapy is often used as a last-ditch effort to control the cancer. Until recently, most chemotherapy has proven very disappointing in its effect on thyroid cancer. Over the last five years, however, a number of new, targeted chemotherapy agents have started to become available.

Although none of these has yet been proven to be effective in treating thyroid cancer, several of them are being actively studied in clinical trials, which are available as an option for patients with thyroid cancer that does not respond to more traditional treatments. These trials are being conducted at a number of large medical centers around the country, and details of all of the currently available clinical trials are available through the National Cancer Institute (www.cancer.gov). Your endocrinologist can arrange a referral to an appropriate trial if necessary.

Case history

Debbie Harris was 18 when she was involved as a passenger in a motor vehicle accident. Fortunately she was wearing her seat belt, but she suffered a whiplash injury, and the seat belt left a lot of bruising across her neck and chest.

As the pain and bruising settled she noticed a small lump in her neck. At first her doctor thought that it must be related to the accident, but the lump moved when she swallowed, suggesting that it lay within the thyroid gland rather than in the skin or muscle. Because the lump was still there after another few weeks, he referred Debbie to an endocrinologist.

Careful examination of Debbie's neck also revealed three enlarged lymph nodes on the right side of her neck. An ultrasound scan confirmed the nodule in her thyroid gland, measuring 1.8 centimeters (about ¾ of an inch), as well as enlarged lymph nodes. He recommended a fine needle aspiration biopsy (FNAB), which was performed with the ultrasound right in the endocrinologist's office. The test took only a few minutes, causing Debbie almost no discomfort and with no need even for a local anesthetic.

The following day, Debbie learned that the lump in her neck was almost certainly a papillary thyroid cancer, which had spread to the nearby lymph nodes, and that the proper treatment was surgery. She met the endocrine surgeon later the same day, and was scheduled for surgery the following week. At that time, her entire thyroid gland was removed, together with the enlarged lymph nodes. She suffered no complications and was sent home from hospital and put on a course of thyroxine medication.

A few weeks later, she met the endocrinologist again, who told her that the cancer was "Stage 1," the earliest possible stage. A detailed ultrasound of the neck proved negative, with no sign of suspicious lymph nodes. The blood test showed that the thyroglobulin level was not detectable and her TSH level was low, just as the endocrinologist had recommended.

After a long discussion of the pros and cons of radioactive iodine treatment, she and her endocrinologist decided that it was not necessary. She was regularly monitored with ultrasound, lab work, and a visit to the endocrinologist every year.

That was ten years ago now, and although she continues to have her lab work checked every year, there has never been any sign of recurrence and she is cured. She continues to take thyroxine, but now keeps her TSH toward the low end of the normal range. Looking back on it now, she sees the accident as a blessing in disguise, because it brought to light a thyroid cancer that was at a very early stage. The fact that it had spread to the lymph nodes in the neck was of no consequence for her long term health.

KEY POINTS

■ Thyroid nodules are common, but thyroid cancer is rare

■ The two most common types of thyroid cancer—papillary and follicular cancers—can normally be treated successfully if they are caught early enough

■ The usual treatment for thyroid cancer of all types is surgery to remove the cancer and all or part of the thyroid gland

■ Some patients at higher than average risk, or in whom complete removal of the cancer could not be achieved, may need treatment with radioactive iodine

■ After surgery, patients will need to take thyroxine in a slightly higher dose than normal, to lower the TSH

■ Follow up will be necessary following surgery to ensure that the cancer has been eliminated and to make sure it does not recur

■ The combination of a thyroglobulin measurement on the blood, ultrasound scan of the neck, and sometimes a whole body iodine scan, are effective ways to follow up most patients with thyroid cancer

■ The prognosis for most patients with thyroid cancer is excellent, with a normal life expectancy. Patients at higher risk from their cancer can usually be identified by staging and risk-scoring at the time of their original diagnosis

Thyroid blood tests

Measuring thyroid hormone levels

Interpretation of thyroid tests can sometimes be confusing, even for doctors. The key to understanding thyroid tests is to remember that TSH is the body's message to the thyroid, calling for more thyroid hormone. If the TSH level is high, this is the body's way of telling the thyroid gland to work harder and indicates that the levels of thyroid hormone are too low. Similarly, if the TSH is low, the body is trying to shut down the thyroid, because the levels of thyroid hormone are too high.

When measuring thyroid hormone levels themselves, it is important to know that most of the thyroid hormone in the blood is bound to other proteins, and is therefore inactive. Of this total amount of hormone, only a tiny fraction—the free hormone—is active.

Nowadays, most labs measure the free thyroxine when they report the T_4 levels. Measurements of T_3 may be of the total or the free hormone. In a few labs, the "T_3-uptake" is used as an indirect method to measure T_3, though this technique has fallen out of favor in recent years because it is less accurate than the direct measurement of T_3. In most circumstances, measurement of free and total thyroid hormones

Normal reference ranges

This table shows the normal reference range of thyroid hormones and TSH in the blood. Your doctor will compare your results with these to assess your condition. Different labs may have slightly different normal range values, depending on the details of the type of test they are using. You should always compare your results to the normal range for the lab performing your tests.

TSH	0.3–5.0 milliunits per liter (mU/L)
Free-T_4	0.8–1.8 nanograms per deciliter (ng/dL)
Free-T_3	2.3–4.2 nanograms per deciliter (ng/dL)
TPO Antibodies	<20 units per liter (U/L)
Total-T_4	5.0–12.5 micrograms/deciliter (mg/dL)
Total-T_3	80–180 nanograms/deciliter (ng/dL)

provide the same information about whether the thyroid is working normally or is over- or underactive.

The normal ranges for TSH, total T_4 (TT_4), free T_4 (fT_4), total T_3 (TT_3) and free T_3 (fT_3) are shown above. Most physicians will request only a few of these tests when assessing patients with thyroid disease.

Of all the tests, the single most accurate test is the TSH test, but it is important to remember that the TSH is not a perfect test. Indeed, all of the testing discussed in this book, including lab work, scans, uptake measurements, and even pathology reports, need to be interpreted in the light of the clinical situation, something that should be done only after a careful history and physical examination has been conducted by a trained doctor.

Remember, also, that normal ranges will vary slightly from laboratory to laboratory, depending on the normal population used for the calculations, and on the type of analysis used for the measurement of the hormones.

Typical results in hyperthyroidism and hypothyroidism
Hyperthyroidism

In most patients with hyperthyroidism, the TSH will be suppressed below the lower end of the normal range, and often the reading is well below the limit of detection, around 0.01mU/L.

The total and free T_4 levels will typically be elevated, and the degree to which they are elevated indicates the severity of the thyroid problem.

In general, people with the worst symptoms will have the highest level of thyroid hormones, but this does not always hold true, because some people seem to be particularly sensitive to changes in thyroid hormone levels.

In addition, even slightly elevated thyroid hormone levels in some older patients can have a very significant adverse effect on their health, if it triggers atrial fibrillation, or exacerbates osteoporosis to the point of causing a fracture.

Hypothyroidism

By the time a patient develops severe symptoms of hypothyroidism fT_4 levels are usually quite low, often less than 0.3 ng/dL.

The TSH will almost always be very high, mostly well above 20 mU/L, and sometimes as high as 80 or 100 mU/L. Young people whose pituitary seems to be particularly strong can drive their TSH level much higher than older people, so the TSH itself is often not a very good marker of how "severe" the hypothyroidism is. An older adult with a TSH of 25 mU/L may be much more severely affected than a young patient with a TSH of over 100 mU/L.

Once again, some people seem to be particularly sensitive to changes of thyroid hormone levels, so that some patients feel symptoms of hypothyroidism even when their TSH is only slightly elevated, while others feel almost nothing at all wrong, even with blood work that makes their physician quake!

Rarely, hypothyroidism is the result of disease of the pituitary gland and not of the thyroid gland itself, in which case the low fT_4 or TT_4 is combined with a normal or low level of TSH. This is a very unusual condition, which requires an assessment by an endocrinologist.

In mild or subclinical hypothyroidism (see page 66), the T_4 level remains in the lower part of the normal range, while the TSH is only modestly elevated, in the region of 5–10 mU/L. The level of T_3 is not usually measured in patients with suspected hypothyroidism.

Adjusting the dose of thyroxine

The goal of treatment with thyroid hormone is to obtain completely normal levels of thyroid hormones and TSH, except for patients with thyroid cancer, in whom a lower than normal TSH might be desired.

Your physician will usually prescribe a starting dose of thyroxine based on your thyroid condition, your age, and body weight. After 6 to 12 weeks, the levels of TSH should be rechecked and the dose adjusted from there as necessary.

For most patients with hypothyroidism, the ideal dose of thyroxine is one that puts the TSH into the normal range. Some patients continue to experience symptoms of mild hypothyroidism, however, unless their TSH is brought down towards the lower end of the normal range, by raising the T_4 toward the upper part of its normal range—in other words, using a slightly higher dose of thyroxine. The target range for TSH should probably be between 0.3 and 2.0 mU/L for these patients.

For a few patients, hypothyroid symptoms can only be eliminated when the T_4 is raised above normal, and the TSH suppressed to below the lower end of the normal range. Many endocrinologists are concerned about possible adverse health consequences of keeping the TSH too low and the T_4 level high, particularly because of the possibility of heart and bone problems. This is particularly a concern amongst older patients, who are at higher risk of developing these complications.

Certainly it is important to consider any possible adverse consequences of this biochemical abnormality, and in this circumstance, it is essential that the T_3 level in the blood is unequivocally normal in order to avoid complications of hyperthyroidism.

Effect of illness on thyroid blood tests

Serious illness of any type, including cancer, heart attack, stroke, rheumatoid arthritis, or depression, can affect the results of thyroid blood tests and lead to a false diagnosis of hyper- or hypothyroidism. It is possible that, after referral to a specialist and after further investigations, no underlying thyroid disease will be found. This is particularly true for thyroid tests performed in the hospital during an admission for some other serious illness. Such tests should be viewed with caution and interpreted by an endocrinologist.

THYROID BLOOD TESTS SHOULD NEVER BE INTERPRETED IN ISOLATION. AN ACCURATE DIAGNOSIS AND APPROPRIATE TREATMENT DEPENDS ON A CAREFUL HISTORY AND PHYSICAL EXAMINATION, WITH BLOOD TESTS AND OTHER EVALUATIONS PROVIDING ADDITIONAL INFORMATION.

KEY POINTS

- The normal ranges for thyroid blood tests will vary from laboratory to laboratory

- In most cases—but not all—the more severe the symptoms the more abnormal the results of the thyroid blood test

- Thyroid blood tests should never be interpreted in isolation

"Hypothyroidism" with normal blood tests

Some patients become convinced that their symptoms, usually of tiredness, fatigue, weight gain, feeling the cold, and "foggy thinking" are caused by hypothyroidism, even when the TSH is normal.

It is very important for the physician to take this possibility seriously, because there are times when the TSH can be misleading, for example in the presence of a pituitary gland problem, or if there is some other serious illness. Generally, these possibilities can be cleared up by checking the levels of T_4 and T_3, along with the TSH.

It is equally important for both patient and doctor to understand that these symptoms, even though they sound a lot like hypothyroidism, could be due to some other problem. The danger is that the thyroid will become so much the focus of attention that other serious underlying conditions might be missed.

This problem has been made worse in recent years

by a number of articles in newspapers, magazines, books, and on the internet in which the authors claim that thyroid disease cannot be diagnosed accurately by modern medical means. They claim that blood tests are inaccurate, and that the diagnosis instead should be made only on the basis of a checklist of symptoms or by measurement of body temperature.

Unfortunately, a small number of practitioners are prepared to diagnose hypothyroidism, and to treat patients with thyroid hormone (often using thyroid hormone extracts), even though the blood tests are normal, or sometimes with no blood testing at all.

Some patients actually start to feel better if they are given thyroid hormone, which reinforces their belief that the problem must lie with the thyroid. The benefit is rarely long-term, however, and certainly does not prove that the problem truly lies with the thyroid. Typically, any benefits are short-lived, and the symptoms return progressively even with continued treatment with thyroid hormone.

I have argued strongly throughout this book that thyroid tests should never be interpreted in isolation— a patient's symptoms and physical findings are always central in making any diagnosis. It is equally false, however, to claim that thyroid blood tests are useless, and that the entire diagnosis should come down to something as silly as a checklist of symptoms, or as inaccurate as the measurement of body temperature.

The following are some common statements and questions from people suffering from symptoms that sound like hypothyroidism, but in whom no other evidence for thyroid disease is found.

"How do you know what level of thyroxine is normal for me?'

The normal range for fT_4 is fairly wide (0.8 to 1.8 ng/mL). If your fT_4 is measured at 1.2 ng/mL, you might ask why it shouldn't be 1.7 or 1.8 ng/mL and whether thyroid hormone should be given to relieve your symptoms. The answer lies in the measurement of the pituitary hormone, TSH, which is your body's way of telling the thyroid (and the treating physician) what level of thyroid hormone it wants to see.

If your "normal" level of fT_4 (say when you were feeling well) was 1.8, but fell to 1.4 because of an undiagnosed thyroid problem, the level of TSH in the blood would rise—well outside the normal range. This would, of course, be an indication that you have a thyroid problem, and should receive treatment with thyroxine. However, if the fT_4 level of 1.2 ng/dL is accompanied by a normal TSH concentration (say 1 or 2 mU/L), this means that your free T_4 concentration is right for you and has been at that level probably for your entire life.

Certainly, the combination of a fT_4 toward the low end of normal (say 0.9 nd/dL) with a high normal TSH, say 4 or 4.5 mU/L, could indicate that you have underlying autoimmune thyroid disease, especially if thyroid antibodies are present in your blood. Most endocrinologists would be willing to treat you with thyroxine, but it would be important not to anticipate a dramatic response, since these levels of thyroid hormone would normally be symptomless or any symptoms would be very mild. Even so, it would be worth treating simply to prevent the onset of more severe hypothyroidism in future years. A few people do gain real and persistent benefits from this treatment, which should certainly be considered for any patient experiencing hypothyroid symptoms, whose hormone studies are borderline or equivocal.

"But I have the symptoms of an underactive thyroid . . ."

The trouble with the symptoms of an underactive thyroid gland is that they are non-specific. Similar symptoms can arise from a wide variety of other medical conditions, or from other events in life. For example, many women in their forties and fifties gain weight and feel tired, as a direct result of the hormonal changes of menopause. Stress at home and at work can lead to sleep disturbance for anyone, as can our increasingly busy and hectic lives. Sleep apnea can often cause disturbed sleep, and may not always present as heavy snoring, or wakening through the night. Sleep deprivation leads to fatigue, tiredness, feeling the cold, weight gain, and aching muscles, as well as memory and problems of "foggy thinking", symptoms that closely resemble those of hypothyroidism.

Other medical conditions can also cause the same type of symptoms: Rheumatoid arthritis causes fatigue, tiredness, and aching just as much as it causes swollen tender joints. Lupus and other chronic inflammatory problems lead to similar symptoms. Depression, which usually makes us feel "low," sometimes masks itself and simply causes fatigue, loss of energy, and sleep disturbance. Some of the symptoms of type II (late onset) diabetes are very similar to those of hypothyroid.

If you have symptoms that sound like thyroid disease, a physical examinations shows that you have features of a thyroid problem, and the lab work confirms a high TSH, low thyroid hormone levels, or both, then there's a pretty good chance that you have a thyroid problem. If you have the same symptoms, but the physical features are missing, or the biochemistry doesn't match, then you and your physician should think very carefully about what else might be going on before starting thyroid hormone.

If you have the right symptoms, but your endocrinologist can't find signs of a thyroid problem and the lab work just doesn't add up, the chance that you have hypothyroidism is very low, and treatment with thyroxine or thyroid hormone extracts are almost certainly not going to be helpful. Treatment with thyroid hormone can have serious complications and side effects if it is used inappropriately. Worse still, treating these symptoms as a thyroid problem may delay or prevent an accurate diagnosis and effective treatment.

"I felt better when I started taking thyroid extract!"

About 20 percent of people given a sugar pill (placebo), believing it to be a real medicine, will feel better no matter what the illness is. This "placebo effect" is a real medical effect, and does not indicate that the person is "weak-willed," stupid, or crazy. It is, in fact, a reminder of just how powerful the mind is in controlling our physical symptoms and sense of well-being.

The placebo effect may last for weeks or months before wearing off. In fact, this experiment has been performed on patients with symptoms that sounded like hypothyroidism, but whose evaluation and blood work was otherwise normal. When these patients were given either the placebo or thyroxine for several weeks, not knowing which they were taking, both groups felt better by about the same degree, and they were unable to tell the difference between the tablets when they were switched. In other words, thyroxine was no better than a placebo.

One additional effect of thyroid hormone, particularly thyroid extract, makes it a commonly used drug in treating patients with non-specific symptoms of this type. Thyroid extract contains quite large amounts of T_3, which is a short and fast-acting hormone. After taking T_3 (in any form), the levels in the blood rise quite rapidly, then fall again, also fairly rapidly. During the rise in T_3, there is an effect on the brain similar to that of caffeine—the recipient gets a buzz or "caffeine boost." Many people drink coffee or caffeinated sodas to gain exactly the same effects—to relieve tiredness and fatigue, boost energy, and sharpen thinking.

Unfortunately, just like those of caffeine, the effects are short-lived. Also like caffeine, the body gradually, but progressively, becomes adapted to the higher levels of T_3, and the benefits slowly but surely wear off. As a result, the temptation is to keep on pushing the dose higher and higher, until toxic side effects—such as palpitations, heart rhythm disturbances, sleep disruption, muscle weakness, and osteoporosis—start to create an equally severe problem.

"What is the harm in taking thyroid hormones if they make me feel better?"

There is no harm for most patients in taking a low dose of thyroxine (say between 50 and 75 mcg daily). Unfortunately, as the "placebo effect" wears off, you and your doctor may be tempted to use higher and higher doses, which will eventually cause symptoms of an overactive thyroid gland. This is even more likely to occur if you are taking a combination of thyroxine and triiodothyronine, or one of the animal thyroid extracts. In the short term, you may be happy with the weight loss and increased energy that comes from hyperthyroidism. In the long term, however, this self-induced hyperthyroidism will lead to significant and troublesome symptoms, including palpitations and possibly diarrhea, loss of muscle mass with a slowed metabolism, and even osteoporosis and possible fracture and to an irregular heartbeat (atrial fibrillation), heart failure, stroke, and even death.

"I know someone who takes both thyroid hormone and steroids because of symptoms like mine"

Addison's disease occurs when the adrenal glands, which sit above the kidneys, fail to produce enough cortisol and other steroid hormones. This disease develops in a few patients with hypothyroidism, because it is also caused by an autoimmune disease. Addison's disease is a serious, potentially life-threatening problem, which requires lifelong use of steroids taken by mouth. It is important to diagnose this condition accurately, and fortunately the test for the disease is very reliable. If you have Addison's disease, you will certainly require steroids, but steroids should never be used to treat a patient who does not require them, and certainly should never be prescribed based on symptoms alone.

So what am I supposed to do about my hypothyroid symptoms, when my TSH is normal?

This can be a very troublesome and distressing group of symptoms, and should be taken seriously. It is not good enough for your physician simply to say: "your TSH is normal" and stop there!

You and your physician need to approach the problem with an open mind, without preconceived ideas of what is and is not the cause. A full, detailed history, a thorough physical examination, and a widespread search for other causes should be undertaken before deciding on a treatment approach. Other hormonal problems, inflammatory and infectious causes, sleep apnea, sleep disruption from other causes, stress, anxiety, and depression should all be considered. In many cases, the problem turns out to be a combination of several such problems, and it certainly would not be surprising if such troublesome symptoms led a person to become stressed or even depressed. Symptoms of this type can easily become self-perpetuating, and—like a whirlpool—they can drag you down.

Treatment should be geared toward the problems that are found, where possible. If the triggers cannot be identified, then treatment should aim at dealing with the symptoms themselves. Just as important as any drug therapy, remember that lifestyle, nutrition, and exercise are important keys to health: good sleep, plenty of exercise, a healthy, well-balanced diet, stress management, good fresh air, a healthy respect for your spiritual needs, and close positive relationships with family and friends.

KEY POINTS

■ Measurements of TSH and T_4 are reliable when interpreted in the light of a detailed history and thorough physical examination, performed by a trained physician

■ Symptoms of hypothyroidism are vague and non-specific, and may be mimicked by many other medical and psychological conditions

■ A patient with symptoms that suggest hypothyroidism, but in whom the physical examination is normal and the hormone levels are also normal almost never benefits long term from thyroid hormone treatment

■ Use of thyroxine or thyroid hormone extracts can give a false sense of improvement, either through a placebo effect, or because of the non-specific "boost" that T_3 has on the brain. The benefits rarely last

■ Thyroid hormone treatment should never be used as a substitute for thorough, thoughtful, and detailed evaluation

Questions and answers

Do I have to change my diet?
Iodine is an integral part of the thyroxine (T_4) and triiodothyronine (T_3) molecules. A lack of iodine in the diet can cause a goiter or hypothyroidism. However, this almost never occurs now in North America because our diet is supplemented with iodine. The current RDA for iodine (150 mcg per day) is enough to ensure normal thyroid health, though pregnant women and nursing mothers may be advised to take more (up to 200 mcg daily). People with a thyroid problem, in particular, should avoid excessive iodine intake, because this can trigger or worsen a pre-existing thyroid condition. Typically, very high levels of iodine are found only in specific supplements, sometimes marketed as thyroid boosters.

Is smoking harmful?
Well, this is a real no-brainer! In the case of thyroid disease, in particular, there is very clear evidence that Graves' Eye Disease is commoner and often more

severe among patients who smoke. So patients with hyperthyroidism caused by Graves' disease have even more reason to stop smoking than everyone else!

Was stress responsible for making my thyroid gland overactive?

Although it is difficult to prove, many endocrinologists are impressed by how often major life events, such as divorce or death of a loved one, have taken place within a few months of the onset of hyperthyroidism caused by Graves' disease. There is evidence that stress can affect the immune system, and it is reasonable to think that this might trigger Graves' disease. So the answer is probably "yes," at least in susceptible people.

Will my new baby have thyroid trouble?

Children born to a mother with Graves' disease—or with a previous history of Graves' disease—may be born with an overactive thyroid gland, called neonatal thyrotoxicosis. This problem generally lasts for only a few weeks and is easily treated.

Occasionally the babies of mothers with hypothyroidism have an underactive thyroid gland at birth. Again this is usually short-lived and will be detected by the routine blood testing of all babies a few days after birth.

Will my children be affected by thyroid disease?

Not necessarily. Although thyroid diseases of several types (Graves' disease, Hashimoto's disease, TMNG, goiter) seem to run in families, the risk to any one individual within a family is usually relatively small. You can get some idea of the risk by looking carefully at your family members. If everyone in the family has a thyroid problem, there's a high chance that your child will develop the problem at some point. Of course, now that you know about it, you can watch for it, and you can have his or her pediatrician check for it periodically if necessary.

Could my thyroid condition explain why I did badly in my college exams?

If hyperthyroidism is not diagnosed and treated, it can certainly affect your concentration and ability to study and retain information. Hypothyroidism can also make it harder to focus, concentrate, and remember. With adequate treatment, these problems should disappear, so you would then have no excuse!

Could thyroid disease have caused my anxiety/depression?

Hyperthyroidism and hypothyroidism can worsen underlying psychiatric problems, but are rarely the main cause of the problem, except in very severe cases. Once again, proper treatment of the thyroid problem will usually eliminate any contribution from the thyroid.

Will my Graves' disease recur?

If your hyperthyroidism has been effectively treated with iodine-131 or surgery, it will almost certainly never return. If the hyperthyroidism settled after a course of antithyroid drugs, there is a 30 to 50 percent chance of recurrence, but this usually happens within one to two years of stopping the drug. After that time, you are much more likely to develop an underactive thyroid, because the immune system may continue to injure and weaken the thyroid gland, causing hypothyroidism.

Does it matter if I forget to take my medication?

The occasional missed dose is not the end of the world. If you discover that you forgot to take your tablet this morning, take it later in the day. If you only realize the following morning, take a double dose—thyroxine is probably the only drug for which you can do this with no ill effects.

For most people, the symptoms of hypothyroidism would not be felt for days or weeks after stopping the tablets altogether. However, missing out tablets is certainly not recommended, because it will lead to less stable thyroid hormone levels, which can themselves cause symptoms. In addition, the TSH and thyroid hormone levels might no longer accurately reflect the dose of thyroid hormone your physician thinks you are taking, leading to inappropriate changes in the prescribed dose of thyroxine. Taking your thyroid hormone regularly, reliably, and appropriately will be well worthwhile in the long run.

I feel better when I am taking a higher dose of thyroxine than recommended by my doctor. Is this safe? There is still some debate about the ideal level of TSH for patients taking thyroxine. The current suggestion is to use enough thyroxine to keep the level of T_4 in the blood at the upper end of the normal range, with the TSH in the lower third of the normal range (between 0.3 and 2.0 mU/L in most labs). Taking too much thyroxine can give you more energy and even help with weight loss in the short term, but there are long-term dangers to the heart and an increased risk of osteoporosis, so this approach is definitely not recommended for most patients.

Will tests involving radioactivity affect my fertility? Definitely not. The amount of radioactivity involved is tiny—less than that in many X-ray tests—so you have no real cause for concern.

Will treatment for Graves' disease make me fat?

No, although you will probably put back on any weight you lost before your thyroid problem was diagnosed. Most people gain some pounds in weight when they are treated, typically 5 to 10 pounds but there's no reason why you should end up weighing any more than you did before you developed Graves' disease. People with very severe Graves' disease may have lost a lot of muscle, which can lead to a slow metabolism—and additional weight gain—once the thyroid is treated. The best way to combat this is to eat right and exercise!

My daughter was put on thyroxine at birth because she was hypothyroid. Will she have to take thyroxine forever?

Not necessarily. Her pediatric endocrinologist may want to stop her thyroxine and then check another blood test when she's about one year old to see whether she still needs the thyroxine. If you had hypothyroidism, it is possible that your daughter's thyroid was just "switched off" by antibodies from your blood stream crossing into hers before and after birth.

Is the time of day when I take my thyroxine tablets important?

It is probably not critical for most people but many of us are best at taking tablets when we develop a regular habit. Thyroxine should be taken on an empty stomach, 30–60 minutes before food, or 3–4 hours after food. No other medication should be taken at the same time—especially not vitamins, minerals, calcium, or iron tablets.

Glossary

This glossary explains the meaning of the most frequently used clinical and related terms connected with the diagnosis and treatment of thyroid disorders.

Anaplastic thyroid cancer: The least common, but most aggressive form of thyroid cancer. This type of cancer often grows rapidly causing pressure symptoms in the neck.

antibodies: these are produced by the body's immune system as a defense mechanism against "foreign" protein contained, for example, in bacteria. Antibodies are not normally formed against proteins that are part of the body. In autoimmune disease, these antibodies can bind to normal tissues and cause problems.

autoimmune disease: antibodies are produced which are directed against normal parts of the body. For example, in most patients with hypothyroidism, antibodies are formed that help to injure the thyroid gland, whereas in Graves' disease antibodies directed against the surface of the thyroid cell stimulate it to over-produce thyroid hormones.

Benign: Non-cancerous, typically used to refer to a thyroid nodule that is present in the gland, but which does not have the potential to spread into other tissues or to the rest of the body.

Carbimazole: One of a group of "anti-thyroid drugs," sometimes used to treat hyperthyroidism. Other members of this group include methimazole (MMZ) and propylthiouracil (PTU).

Cancer: A group of diseases in which abnormal cells divide and grow, forming a "tumor" (swelling), and then invade surrounding tissues, with the potential to spread into surrounding lymph nodes or into most distant parts of the body (metastases).

Cold nodule: A nodule within the thyroid that does not absorb iodine efficiently, and therefore appears "cold" on scanning with radioactive tracers. Although most cancers form cold nodules, most cold nodules turn out to be benign.

de Quervain's thyroiditis: a form of thyroid inflammation that can occur following a viral infection of the thyroid.

Endocrinologist: A specialist in the diagnosis and treatment of diseases of the endocrine system, or glands, including thyroid, adrenal, pituitary and pancreas glands.

euthyroid: a term for normal thyroid function.

exophthalmos: prominence or bulging of the eyes most commonly found in patients with hyperthyroidism caused by Graves' disease. The exophthalmos may affect one or both eyes, may be apparent before the overactive thyroid gland develops and may appear for the first time after successful treatment of the hyperthyroidism.

fine needle aspiration (FNA): a biopsy that involves passing a small needle into the thyroid gland and extracting (aspirating) a small sample of tissue for examination under the microscope. This technique is useful to diagnose the cause of thyroid nodules and goiter.

Follicular thyroid cancer: A cancer of the thyroid which tends to develop in middle-age or older adults, and which can invade into surrounding tissues, or spread elsewhere in the body. This type of cancer carries a prognosis that is much better than Anaplastic thyroid cancer, but not quite as good as the more common Papillary cancer.

goiter: an enlarged thyroid gland, sometimes visible in the neck.

Graves' disease: the name given to the most common form of hyperthyroidism. Patients often have exophthalmos, a goiter, and may have raised red patches on the legs known as pretibial myxedema.

Hashimoto's thyroiditis: the name given to a particular cause of hypothyroidism, in which an underactive thyroid is seen along with a goiter is caused by autoimmune thyroid disease. The term is sometimes used to describe autoimmune thyroid disease, when antibodies are present in the blood, whether or not there is a goiter or hypothyroidism.

Hormone: A chemical substance produced by one of the glands in the body, which is released into the bloodstream. The hormone then acts elsewhere to control or regulate body functions.

Hot nodule: A thyroid nodule that takes up iodine, and which is therefore "hot" on scans performed with radioactive tracers. Hot nodules can cause hyperthyroidism.

hyperthyroidism: condition caused by an overactive thyroid gland, producing too much thyroid hormone.

hypothyroidism: condition caused by underactive thyroid gland, not producing enough thyroid hormone.

iodine: An essential dietary micronutrient. Iodine is found naturally in seafood, shellfish, and seaweed, and at much lower levels in dairy products. In the US, iodine is added to salt and flour, so that iodine deficiency is now very rare.

Lobectomy: Removal of half of the thyroid, often used to treat benign thyroid nodules.

Lymph node: A small mass of lymphatic tissue, surrounded by a capsule. The lymph nodes form part of the lymphatic system, which drain fluid from all parts of the body. These nodes are important in fighting infection, and can also trap cancerous cells. Papillary thyroid cancer is particularly likely to spread to lymph nodes in the neck, where the disease can be trapped and sometimes contained.

Malignant: Cancerous.

Metastasis: Cancer that has spread from its original site to involve another organ of the body. These cancer deposits are sometimes called "secondaries."

methimazole (MMZ): one of the drugs used in the USA to treat hyperthyroidism. It blocks the production of thyroid hormone.

myxedema: this term can be used interchangeably with hypothyroidism, but is often used to describe patients in whom the hypothyroidism is severe and long-standing.

nodule: a lump or swelling, in this case of the thyroid gland. These are mostly benign, but can occasionally be caused by thyroid cancer.

Papillary thyroid cancer: The most common form of thyroid cancer, and usually the most treatable.

parathyroid gland: four parathyroid glands lie on the back of the thyroid, in most people. These glands control the level of calcium in the blood. If they are injured or removed at the time of thyroid surgery, the calcium level can fall, causing tetany.

pituitary gland: This "master gland" lies beneath the brain, behind the bridge of the nose. It regulates most of the glands in the body, including the thyroid gland, which it controls by producing TSH.

postpartum thyroiditis: a temporary disturbance in the balance of the thyroid gland which can occur in the first year after childbirth. There are often no symptoms, but hyperthyroidism and hypothyroidism can both occur. Treatment is not usually necessary.

propranolol (Inderal™): a drug belonging to the group known as beta-blockers which can ease some of the symptoms of hyperthyroidism. Other members of the group include atenolol (Tenormin™) and metoprolol (Toprol™).

proptosis: another word for exophthalmos.

propylthiouracil (PTU): one of the drugs used in the USA to treat hyperthyroidism. It blocks the production of thyroid hormone.

radioactive iodine (iodine-131; I-131): a radioactive isotope of iodine, used in the investigation and treatment of hyperthyroidism.

remnant ablation (radioactive iodine ablation): treatment with radioactive iodine designed to eliminate remnants of normal thyroid tissue, left behind at the time of surgery. This treatment may be useful to decrease the chance of tumor recurrence, for patients with high risk thyroid cancer.

Stage: A way of describing the spread of cancer. Cancer of the thyroid is split into four stages, with stage 1 being the earliest and stage 4 being the most advanced stage.

tetany: this results from a low level of calcium in the blood with tingling in the hands, feet, and around the mouth, and painful spasm of the muscles of the hands and feet.

thyroglobulin: a protein produced by the thyroid gland. Its measurement in the blood is an important part of the follow-up of patients with thyroid cancer.

thyroid function tests: a series of blood tests performed in most labs, looking at the functioning of the thyroid gland. The TSH is the single most accurate thyroid test, but measurements of T_4, T_3, and thyroid antibodies can also provide useful information about diseases of the thyroid gland.

thyroidectomy: surgical removal of all, or part of, the thyroid gland

thyroid stimulating hormone (TSH): a hormone secreted by the pituitary gland, which is responsible for controlling the output of thyroid hormones by the thyroid gland. In hypothyroidism caused by disease of the thyroid gland, TSH concentrations are elevated in the blood, while in hyperthyroidism TSH concentrations are low.

thyrotoxicosis: another term for hyperthyroidism.

thyroxine (T$_4$): a hormone secreted by the thyroid gland, along with triiodothyronine (T$_3$). It has to be converted to T$_3$ in the body before it becomes active. Thyroxine is available in tablet form for the treatment of hypothyroidism.

triiodothyronine (T$_3$): a hormone secreted by the thyroid gland, along with thyroxine. It helps control the body's metabolism. Although it is available in tablet form, it is not usually prescribed for patients with hypothyroidism because it does not provide such good control as thyroxine.

Tumor: An abnormal swelling caused by growth of cells within an organ. Thyroid tumors are usually called "nodules"; most are benign but a few turn out to be cancerous.

ultrasound scan: a scan that uses high frequency sound waves to create images of body structures beneath the skin. This technique is particularly useful to take pictures of the thyroid gland.

Useful addresses

Where can I learn more?

We have included the following organizations because, on preliminary investigation, they may be of use to the reader. However, we do not have firsthand experience of each organization and so cannot guarantee the organization's integrity. The reader must therefore exercise his or her own discretion and judgment when making further inquiries.

Resources specific to thyroid conditions

American Association of Clinical Endocrinologists
Address: 1000 Riverside Avenue, Suite 204,
Jacksonville FL 32204
Tel: 904 353 7878
Fax: 904 353 8185
Website: www.aace.com

American Thyroid Association
Address: 6066 Leesburg Pike, Suite 550, Falls Church,
VA 22041
Tel: 703 998-8890
Fax: 703 998-8893
Website: www.thyroid.org

Johns Hopkins University
The Ripken Program
http://thyroid-ripken.med.jhu.edu/index.html

Mayo Clinic
Address: 200 First Street SW, Rochester, MN 55905
Tel: 507 284-2511
Website: www.mayoc.edu
www.mayoclinic.com

Mount Sinai Hospital, Toronto
Address: 600 University Avenue, Toronto, Canada
M5G 1X5
Tel: 416 596-4200
Website: www.mtsinai.on.ca

National Cancer Institute
Address: Suite 625, 1700 Diagonal Road, Alexandria,
VA 22314
Tel: 703 837-1500
Website: www.cancer.gov
www.nhpco.org

Thyroid Foundation of America
One Longfellow Place, Suite 1518
Boston, MA 02114
Tel: (800) 832-8321
Website: www.tsh.org

General information resources
Freedom From Smoking® Online
www.ffsonline.org

American Lung Association's free online smoking
cessation program.

Healthfinder®
www.healthfinder.gov

A consumer health information website sponsored by the United States government. A resource for finding government and nonprofit health information on the internet.

MayoClinic
www.mayoclinic.com

On-line health information for the layperson

National Health Information Center (NHIC)
P O Box 1133
Washington, DC 20013
U.S.A.
Tel: (800) 336-4797
www.health.gov/NHIC

NHIC, part of the Department of Health and Human Services, helps people locate information on health issues through referral to organizations that can best answer their questions.

U.S. Department of Health and Human Services
200 Independence Avenue, S.W.
Washington, D.C. 20201
Tel: (202) 619-0257
Helpline: (877) 696-6775
www.hhs.gov

Government agency giving information and advice on sickness and disability benefits for people with disabilities and their caregivers.

WebMD
www.webMD.com

On-line health information for the layperson

The internet as a source of further information

After reading this book, you may feel that you would like further information on the subject. The internet is an excellent place to look and many websites contain useful information about medical conditions, related charities, and support groups.

It should always be remembered, however, that the internet is unregulated and anyone is free to set up a website and add information to it. Many websites offer impartial advice and information that has been compiled and checked by qualified medical professionals. Some, on the other hand, are run by commercial organizations with the purpose of promoting their own products. Others still are run by pressure groups, and special interest groups, some of which will provide carefully assessed and accurate information whereas others may be suggesting medications or treatments that are not supported by the medical and scientific community.

Unless you know the address of the website you want to visit—for example, www.webmd.com—you may find the following guidelines useful when searching the internet for information.

Search engines and other searchable sites

Google (www.google.com) is the most popular search engine used in the United States, followed by Yahoo! (www.yahoo.com) and MSN (www.msncom). Also popular are the search engines provided by Internet Service Providers such as AOL (www.aol.com).

In addition to the search engines that index the whole of the web, there are also medical sites with search facilities, which act almost like mini-search engines, covering only medical topics or even a particular area of medicine. Again, it is wise to look at who is responsible for compiling the information offered to ensure that it is impartial and medically accurate.

Search phrases

Be specific when entering a search phrase. Searching for information on "cancer" will return results for many different types of cancer as well as on cancer in general. You may even find sites offering astrological information! More useful results will be returned by using search phrases such as "lung cancer" and "treatments for lung cancer." Both Google and Yahoo offer an advanced search option that includes the ability to search for the exact phrase; enclosing the search phrase in quotes, that is, "treatments for lung cancer," will have the same effect. Limiting a search to an exact phrase reduces the number of results returned but it is best to refine a search to an exact match only if you are not getting useful results with a normal search.

Always remember the internet is international and unregulated. It holds a wealth of valuable information but individual sites may be biased, out-of-date, or just plain wrong. Family Doctor Publications accepts no responsibility for the content of links published in this series.

Index

Your pages

We have included the following pages because they may help you manage your illness or condition and its treatment.

Before an appointment with a health professional, it can be useful to write down a short list of questions about anything you don't understand, so that you can make sure that you don't forget anything.

Some of the sections may not be relevant to your circumstances.

Health-care contact details

Name:

Practitioner type:

Place of work:

Tel:

Name:

Practitioner type:

Place of work:

Tel:

Name:

Practitioner type:

Place of work:

Tel:

Name:

Practitioner type:

Place of work:

Tel:

**Significant past health events—illnesses/
operations/investigations/treatments**

Event	Month	Year	Age (at time)

Appointments for health care

Name:

Place:

Date:

Time:

Tel:

Name:

Place:

Date:

Time:

Tel:

Name:

Place:

Date:

Time:

Tel:

Name:

Place:

Date:

Time:

Tel: